HARROW COLLEGE
HH Learning Centre
Lowlands Road, Harrow
Middx HA1 3AQ
020 8909 6520

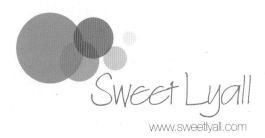

Sweet Lyall

the
asian bridal
look book

dedicated to our families

First published January 2005 by Buzzword UK
on behalf of Sweet Lyall Ltd
www.buzzworduk.com
www.sweetlyall.com tel: 0871 990 7721

Copyright © Sweet Lyall Ltd

ISBN 1-902544-06-4

A CIP record for this title is available from the
British Library

Printed by MWL Print Group
South Wales, UK

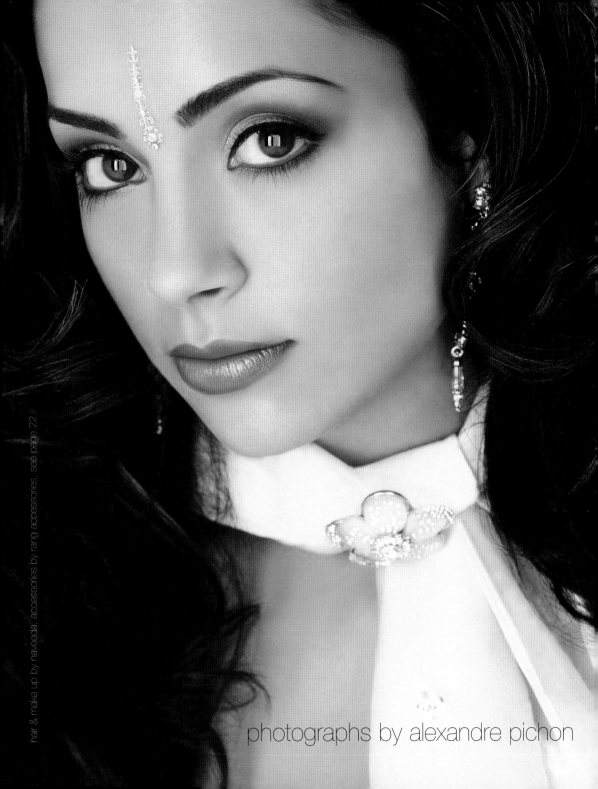

photographs by alexandre pichon

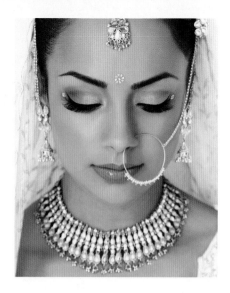

"Brimming with all things bride and beautiful, this book will prove invaluable to any woman wanting to look her best on her wedding day."

Shihab Salim, Editor-in-Chief, Asiana Wedding

Cover Credits

Hair & Make-up: Nina Haider
Outfit: Khubsoorat
Accessories & Bindis: Bombay Looks
Broach in Hair: Rang Accessories

Back Cover Credits

Hair & Make-up: Naveeda
Outfit: Rang Collection
Accessories & Bindis: Bombay Looks

For further information on forthcoming titles,
please refer to www.sweetlyall.com

the
asian bridal
look book

concept: kiran lyall

creative director & editor: nilpa bharadia

art director & design: venisha padhiar

photography: alexandre pichon

hair & make-up design: naveeda & nina haider

additional hair & make-up: monique lagnerius

stylist: navreet jhutti

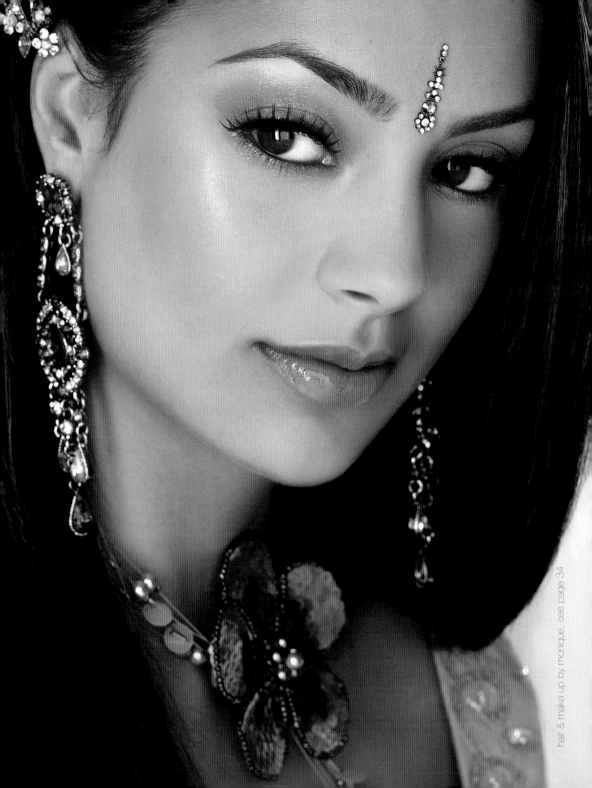

contents

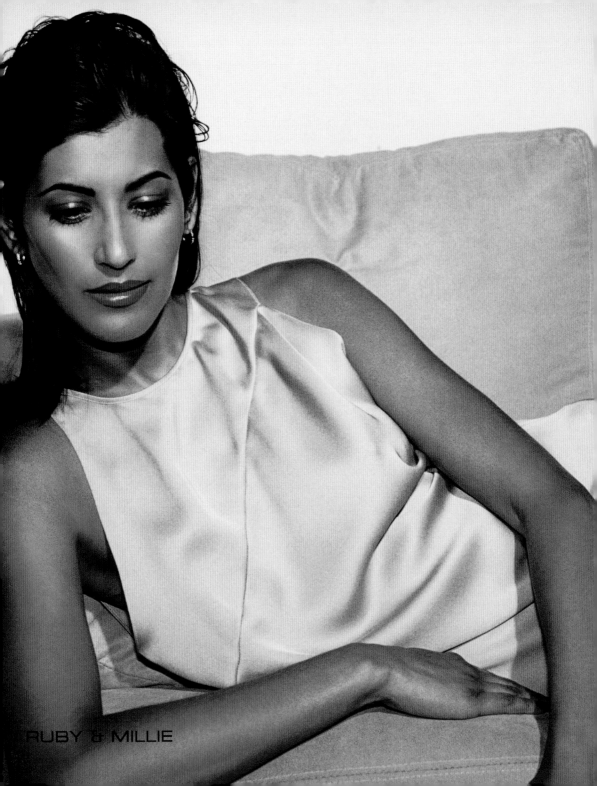

RUBY & MILLIE

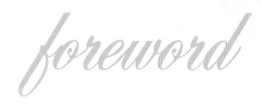

ruby hammer

My unending love affair and passion for make-up goes right back to my childhood. The inspiration for this is none other than my beautiful and glamorous mother. She was the epitome of grace and beauty, and to me as stunning as any Bollywood film heroine. Leaning on her dressing table I would study her as she applied her lotions and potions, colours and creams, mesmerising me as I was transported away watching her change before my very eyes.

My inspiration ended up taking me to my career path, a path that has been riddled with reoccurring questions: how does one find the best 'look'? How can it be adapted to have a low key effect or really up the drama factor? Which colours will suit me? These dilemmas and others like them are applicable to all women irrespective of colour, race or age. For Asian woman there are the added difficulties in finding a look or products that suit their particular skin tone. It's a fact that Asian skins are not largely catered for in the mass market place, however this situation has improved slightly today with the launch of brands such as MAC and Ruby & Millie to name but a few. Despite this, Asian women still appear to be confused and unsure as to what they should be going for. Mainstream magazines do offer a variety of hints and tips, but are these ultimately going to benefit them?

Asian women also have another unique need. Culturally they face more opportunities for dressing up - weddings, religious events and all manner of socialising are part of their everyday lives. The Asian lady tends to dress up rather than down, and her clothes are colourful and rich, vibrant and varied, and this is never truer than for a bride.

Brides need to be stunning, not only for their wedding, but also for all the events leading up to the big day. Apart from the clothes there is intricate and elaborate jewellery to contend with and a bride's beauty needs to blossom and radiate through all of this outer and sometimes over-consuming costume. A daunting prospect especially when they know that any mistakes will be captured forever on film.

So its vital that any woman trying to make the most of her looks will have to be prepared to experiment with new colours, products and tools. Thankfully this book allows you to do just this in your own time and the privacy of your home. It is such a godsend, not only to brides, but also for all Asian women who need occasion make-up in their lives, and let's face it; there are loads of them.

I hope you will enjoy using this book as a guide to enable yourself to gain confidence to really go for it, whatever the occasion. Enjoy!

Best Wishes,

Ruby x

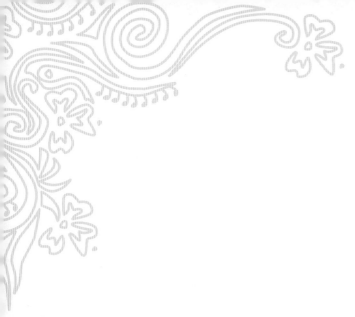

a brief message...

Fate is a game of numbers and possibility; in life you will come across numerous paths that will lead you to another stage in your journey, be that getting married or creating a book that will inspire that very bride to be. Ours is the story of the latter. Conceived on a rainy platform in East London no less, Kiran and I created The Asian Bridal Look Book. Out of the 100's of ideas that kept swimming around in our heads, this one kept trying to stalk our consciences until we could no longer ignore it.

After working on one of the countries biggest Asian bridal magazines, we decided to walk away from the careers that we had both spent a combined total of fifteen years developing. Hopefully the decision to make a change in our lives was justified. If not, then please excuse us for being self-indulgent.

We both whole heartedly believe in this book and the power of good it will do for all Asian women who want to look gorgeous on their special day. Don't get us wrong, it's not going to clear your credit cards or help you loose twenty pounds, but what we can promise is that it will stop you from making a huge beauty faux pas. With the help of this book, you will be able to look back on your special day without wincing, safe in the knowledge that you got it right.

Getting it right is the holy grail of every bride-to-be's existence. Your make-up ranks as one of the most important decisions to do with your overall look. After all, you can spend thousands on a beautiful bespoke outfit, but if your face looks like it has been dipped in atta, then lets face it, no one is going to be admiring your thread-work.

Make-up can mean a lot of different things to Asian women. To some its an essential armour against the trials and tribulations of life, whilst to others it's a glass alarm - do not smash unless in cases of an emergency. But when you get married, it really is a situation of there is nowhere left to run, no sunglasses to hide behind or no trowel big enough to shovel it on. Any mistake will ultimately be a 'huge' mistake, which sadly, will be immortalised for your displeasure on your wedding photographs.

introduction

Not that, that means you should start thinking about consigning yourself to a life of only cats for companions, for fear of sending him running in the opposite direction upon glimpse of your ill made up face. Rest assured help is at hand; cue The Asian Bridal Look Book, its not clad in lycra tights, but is filled with a 150 pages of ideas and inspiration that will put an end to your world destruction in minutes. It is the salvation that you have been looking for – hail your very own beauty bible.

Our aim is to equip you with some of the best beauty looks that money can buy on a budget, supplied by your very own celebrity make-up artists. These wonder women, are armed with lip brushes, and have specially been chosen to make sure you look like a vision of co-ordinated beauty on your wedding day.

It's as simple as flicking through the book to find the page that has the colour of your outfit on it and then discovering a beautifully created look next to it. Once you've decided on what shade suits you best, then find a perfectly coffered hairstyle to complement it. In short you too have the chance to look as gorgeous as the film, television and pop stars that these make up artists have worked on.

No longer will you have to visit your own beautician and sit nervously through the consultation like it's a visit to the dentist. Instead carry your very own handy sized beauty bible to your girlfriends and pore over the looks together. You can take it shopping with you when you pick that all-important outfit or simply read it on the tube on the way to work. Knowledge most certainly is power and confidence. Sure you'll need a little bit of bravery for good measure, but once you've realised that there is more to bridal beauty than maroon lipstick and thick eyeliner, you'll be able to open your eyes to an infinite number of tailor made looks... remember, its all a game of numbers, pick your lucky one.

Good luck

Nilpa, Editor

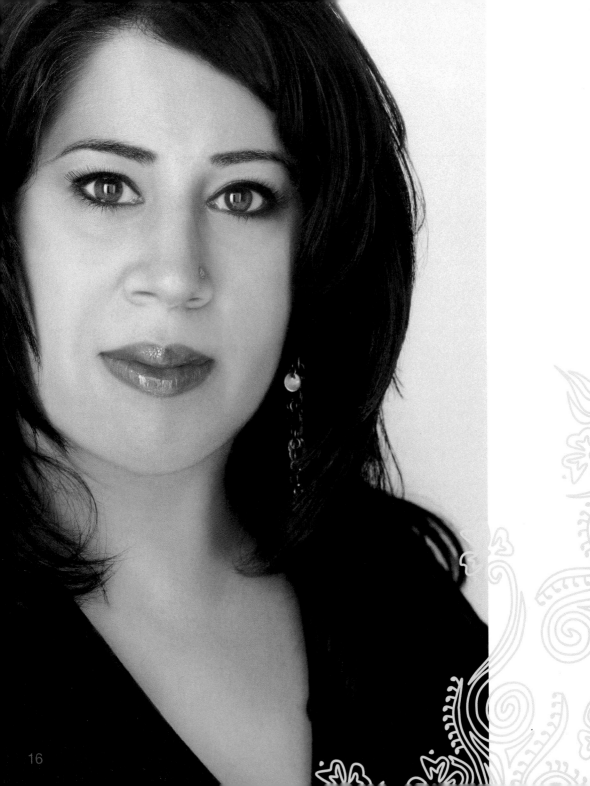

16

" I like to think that I'm in the business of making women from all walks of life feel wonderful. To me make-up is much more than applying lipstick, it's about applying confidence, and that's one of the greatest gifts you can give to another woman."

naveeda

Often credited for turning the ordinary into the extraordinary, Naveeda has a gift for transforming her subjects with the simple stroke of a brush. In a competitive industry where many have tried and failed she is an exceptional success story, having established herself firmly as an innovative leading bridal make-up professional.

A qualified hair & make-up artist, she is also a very successful beauty therapist. Loved by her clients and veneered by her peers, she has managed to create a signature style, which is both quintessential and imaginative,

Trained by a BBC make-up artist, she has since become a highly sought after individual in her own right. Today, she is the first name in every Asian magazine Editor's contact book, as her regular contribution on leading bridal and fashion bibles such as Asiana, Asiana Wedding, Asian Bride and Asian Woman shows.

Aside from being a magazine cover veteran, her work has also graced other famous canvases, from beauty queen Farheen Khan, to celebrities like film and TV star Laila Rouass. International dignitaries and companies such as Universal Records have also acknowledged her work.

Her genuine warmth and amazing talent assures that she will continue to be one of the countries leading make-up artists for many years to come.

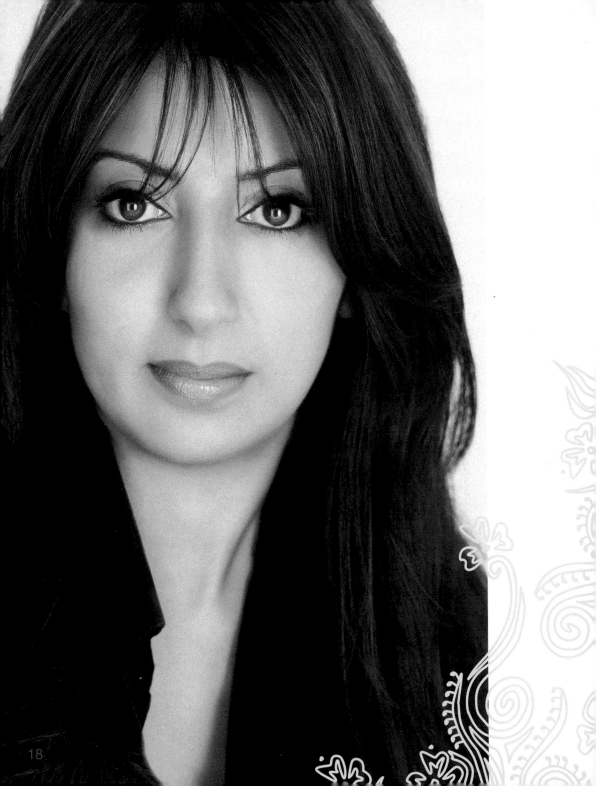

" My professional philosophy has always been simple. I've always believed that make-up should enhance a woman's natural beauty rather than create another face."

nina haider

Nina Haider first discovered her flair for make-up through her love of art. Her talents with a paint brush led her to master her skills to greater effect when she swapped her acrylic paints for lipsticks and eyeshadow's in adult life.

A fully certified hair & make-up artist and beauty therapist, she was determined to carve out a name for herself. She spent years developing her trade working for some of the worlds best known cosmetic houses, such as Estee Lauder and Christian Dior. It wasn't long before she was being pursued by the likes of Chanel, who even gave her, her own beauty room, at one of London's most prestigious stores.

Her success with clients enabled Nina to branch out on her own and create a reputation that is now formidable. Considered to be a pioneer of make-up styles, her mark can clearly be seen in bridal looks today. These looks have inspired a generation of brides to break the boundaries of fashion make-up and pursue new ways of enhancing their beauty.

Her portfolio is also filled with a who's who of Asian celebrities. When Meera Syal and Parminder Nagra had premiere's of their films to attend, Nina was their first choice. When Shobna Gulati's character in 'Coronation Street,' was getting married, she naturally turned to Nina.

With magazine covers, fashion spreads, London Fashion Week, and clients like Radox and M&S, Nina has most certainly put the 'art' into make-up artist.

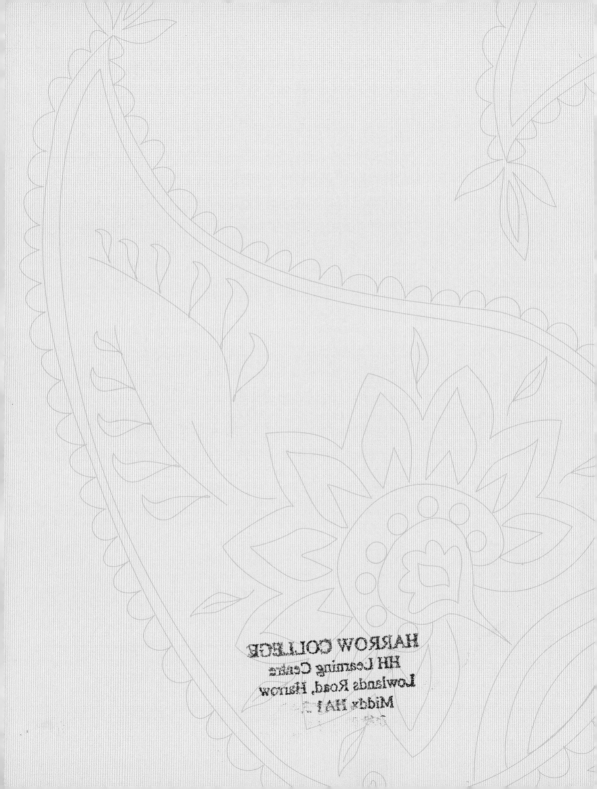

7

contemporary looks

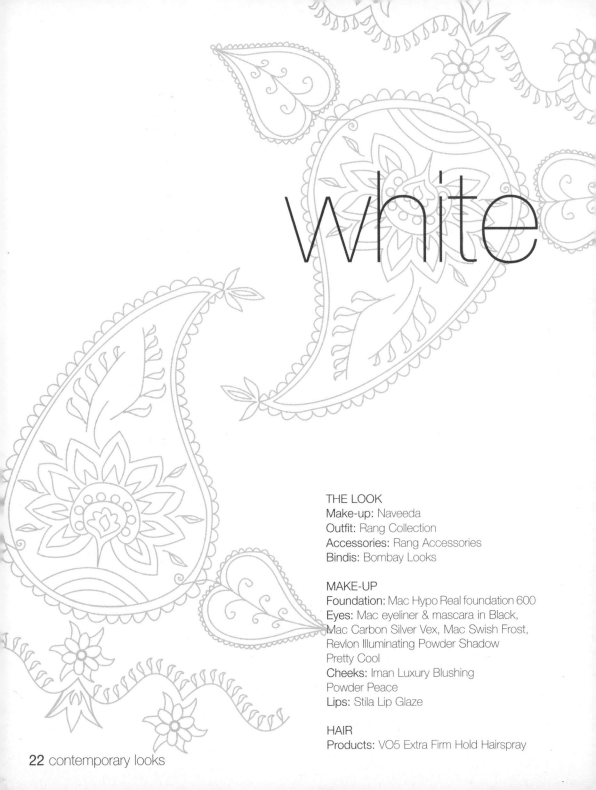

white

THE LOOK
Make-up: Naveeda
Outfit: Rang Collection
Accessories: Rang Accessories
Bindis: Bombay Looks

MAKE-UP
Foundation: Mac Hypo Real foundation 600
Eyes: Mac eyeliner & mascara in Black,
Mac Carbon Silver Vex, Mac Swish Frost,
Revlon Illuminating Powder Shadow
Pretty Cool
Cheeks: Iman Luxury Blushing
Powder Peace
Lips: Stila Lip Glaze

HAIR
Products: VO5 Extra Firm Hold Hairspray

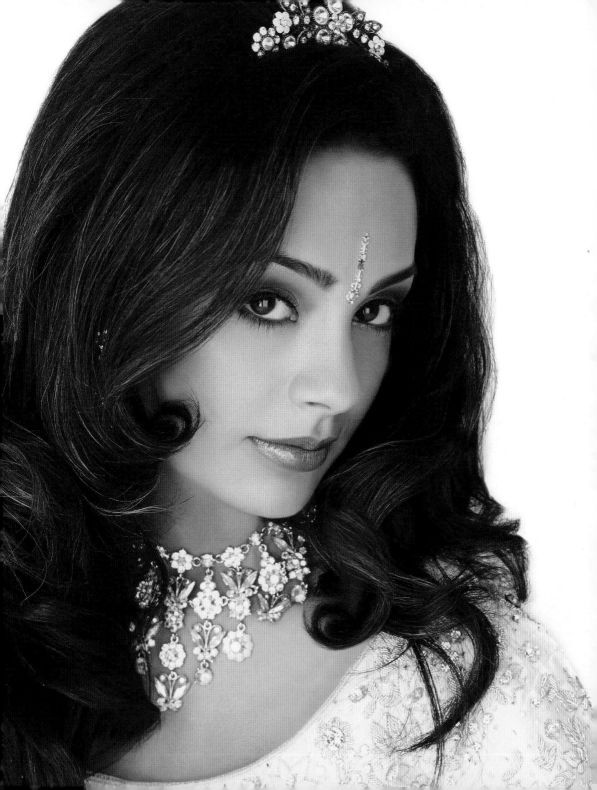

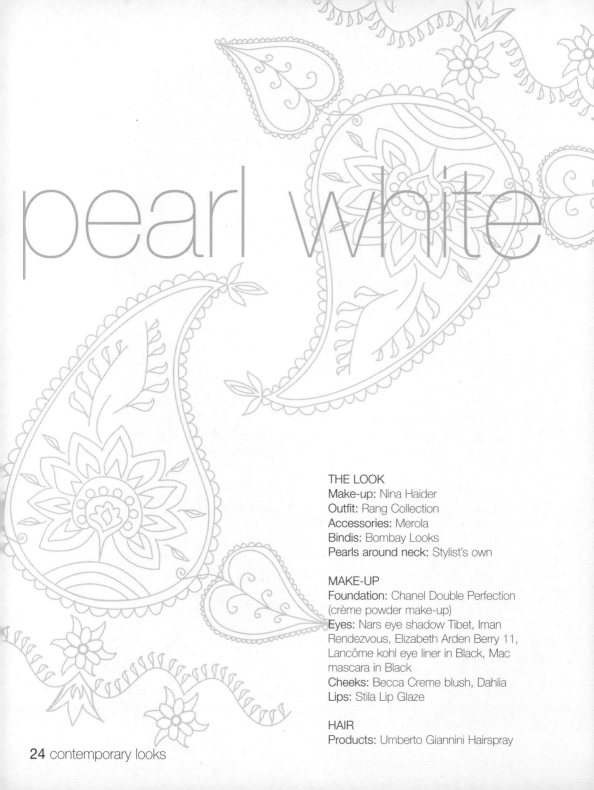

pearl white

THE LOOK
Make-up: Nina Haider
Outfit: Rang Collection
Accessories: Merola
Bindis: Bombay Looks
Pearls around neck: Stylist's own

MAKE-UP
Foundation: Chanel Double Perfection (crème powder make-up)
Eyes: Nars eye shadow Tibet, Iman Rendezvous, Elizabeth Arden Berry 11, Lancôme kohl eye liner in Black, Mac mascara in Black
Cheeks: Becca Creme blush, Dahlia
Lips: Stila Lip Glaze

HAIR
Products: Umberto Giannini Hairspray

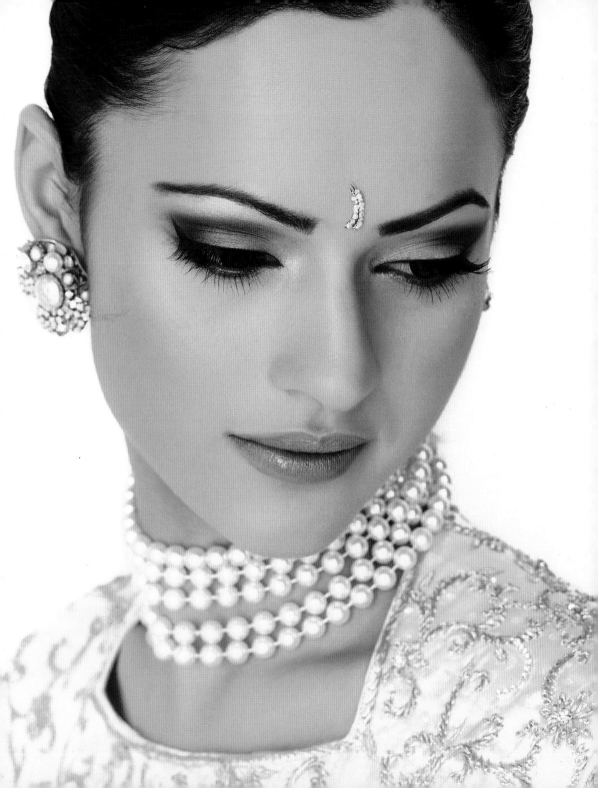

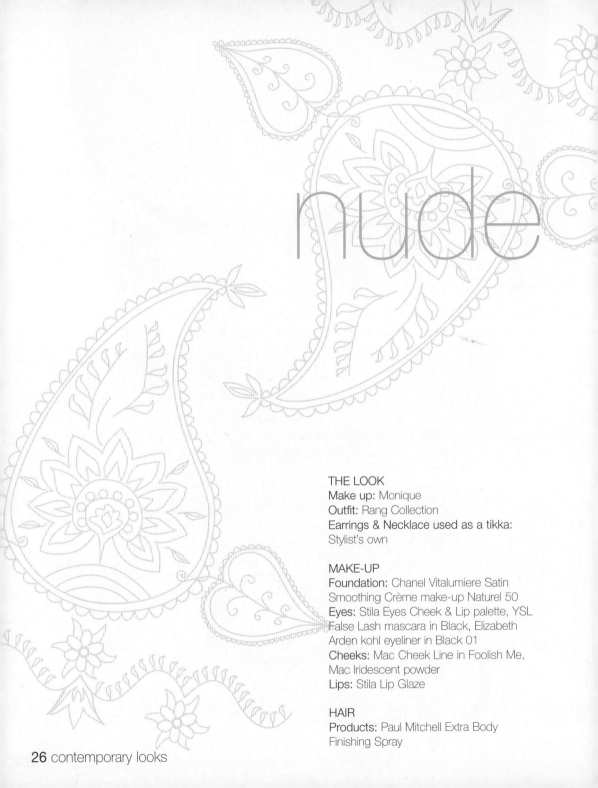

nude

THE LOOK
Make up: Monique
Outfit: Rang Collection
Earrings & Necklace used as a tikka:
Stylist's own

MAKE-UP
Foundation: Chanel Vitalumiere Satin
Smoothing Crème make-up Naturel 50
Eyes: Stila Eyes Cheek & Lip palette, YSL
False Lash mascara in Black, Elizabeth
Arden kohl eyeliner in Black 01
Cheeks: Mac Cheek Line in Foolish Me,
Mac Iridescent powder
Lips: Stila Lip Glaze

HAIR
Products: Paul Mitchell Extra Body
Finishing Spray

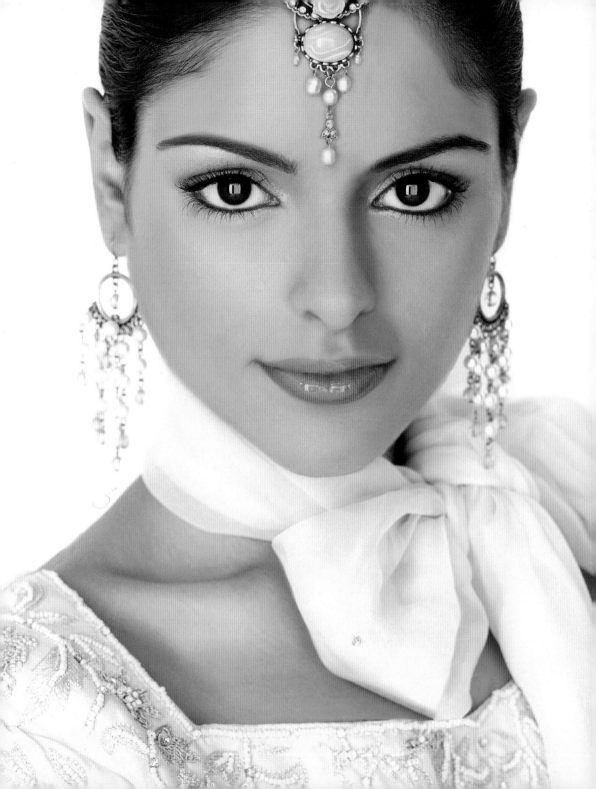

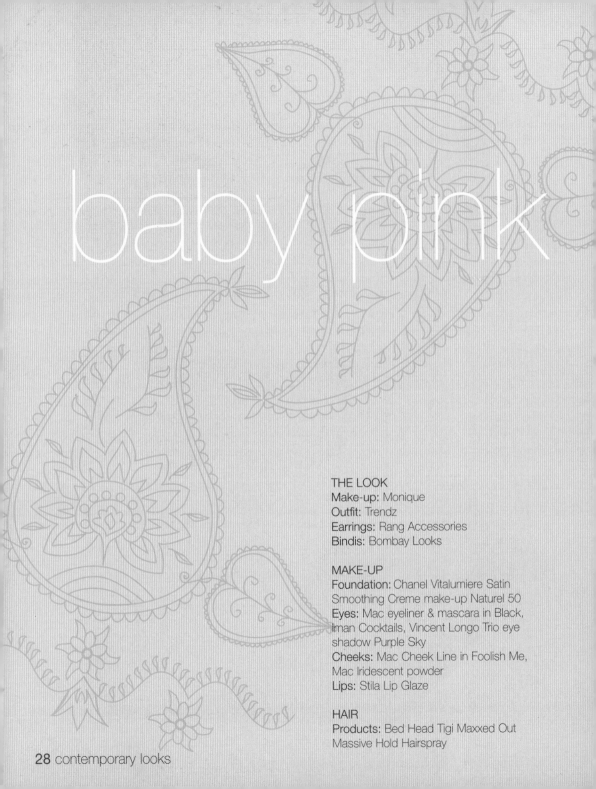

baby pink

THE LOOK
Make-up: Monique
Outfit: Trendz
Earrings: Rang Accessories
Bindis: Bombay Looks

MAKE-UP
Foundation: Chanel Vitalumiere Satin
Smoothing Creme make-up Naturel 50
Eyes: Mac eyeliner & mascara in Black,
Iman Cocktails, Vincent Longo Trio eye
shadow Purple Sky
Cheeks: Mac Cheek Line in Foolish Me,
Mac Iridescent powder
Lips: Stila Lip Glaze

HAIR
Products: Bed Head Tigi Maxxed Out
Massive Hold Hairspray

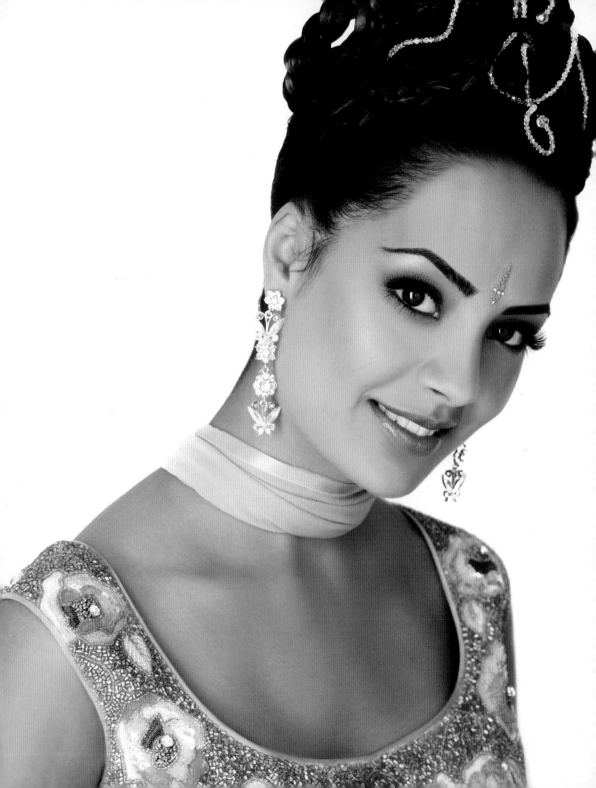

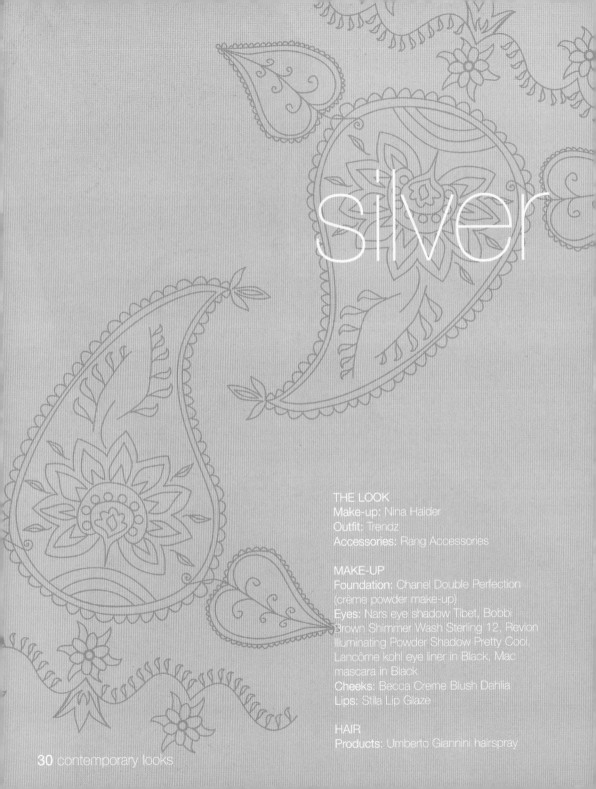

silver

THE LOOK
Make-up: Nina Haider
Outfit: Trendz
Accessories: Rang Accessories

MAKE-UP
Foundation: Chanel Double Perfection
(creme powder make-up)
Eyes: Nars eye shadow Tibet, Bobbi
Brown Shimmer Wash Sterling 12, Revlon
Illuminating Powder Shadow Pretty Cool,
Lancôme kohl eye liner in Black, Mac
mascara in Black
Cheeks: Becca Creme Blush Dahlia
Lips: Stila Lip Glaze

HAIR
Products: Umberto Giannini hairspray

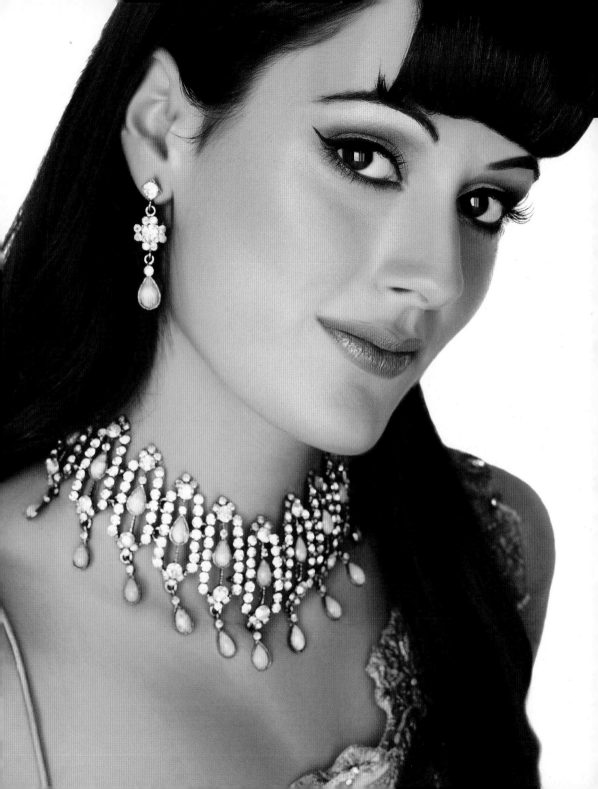

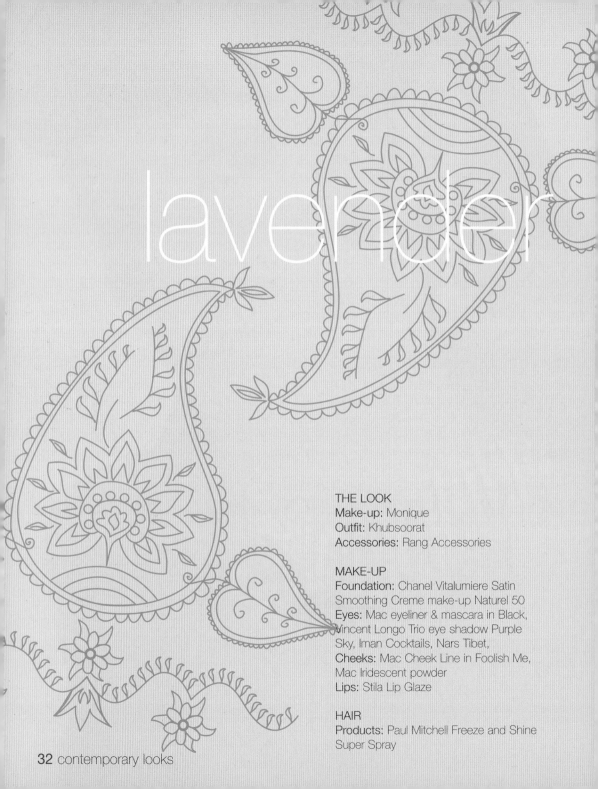

lavender

THE LOOK
Make-up: Monique
Outfit: Khubsoorat
Accessories: Rang Accessories

MAKE-UP
Foundation: Chanel Vitalumiere Satin
Smoothing Creme make-up Naturel 50
Eyes: Mac eyeliner & mascara in Black,
Vincent Longo Trio eye shadow Purple
Sky, Iman Cocktails, Nars Tibet,
Cheeks: Mac Cheek Line in Foolish Me,
Mac Iridescent powder
Lips: Stila Lip Glaze

HAIR
Products: Paul Mitchell Freeze and Shine
Super Spray

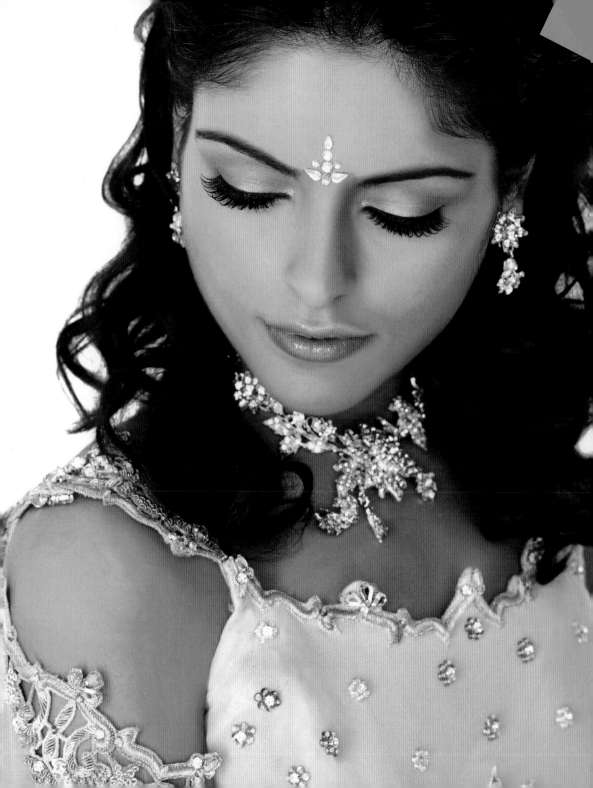

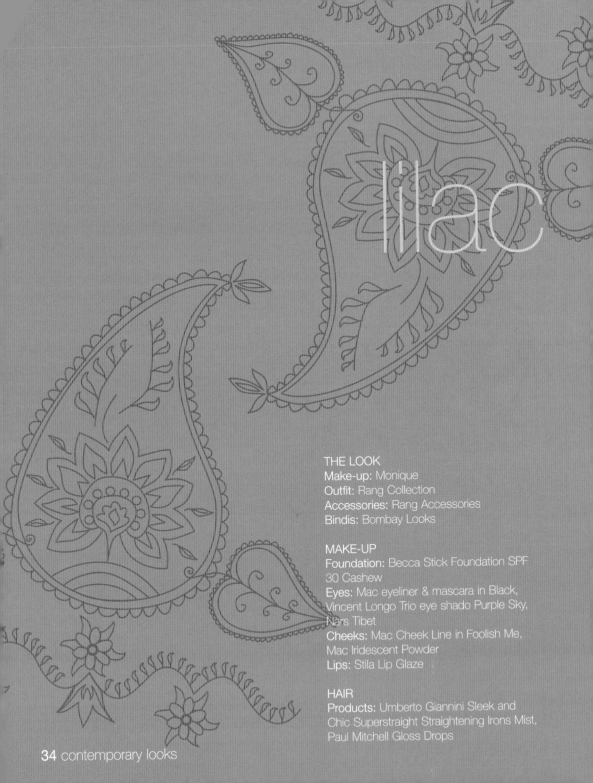

lilac

THE LOOK
Make-up: Monique
Outfit: Rang Collection
Accessories: Rang Accessories
Bindis: Bombay Looks

MAKE-UP
Foundation: Becca Stick Foundation SPF 30 Cashew
Eyes: Mac eyeliner & mascara in Black, Vincent Longo Trio eye shado Purple Sky, Nars Tibet
Cheeks: Mac Cheek Line in Foolish Me, Mac Iridescent Powder
Lips: Stila Lip Glaze

HAIR
Products: Umberto Giannini Sleek and Chic Superstraight Straightening Irons Mist, Paul Mitchell Gloss Drops

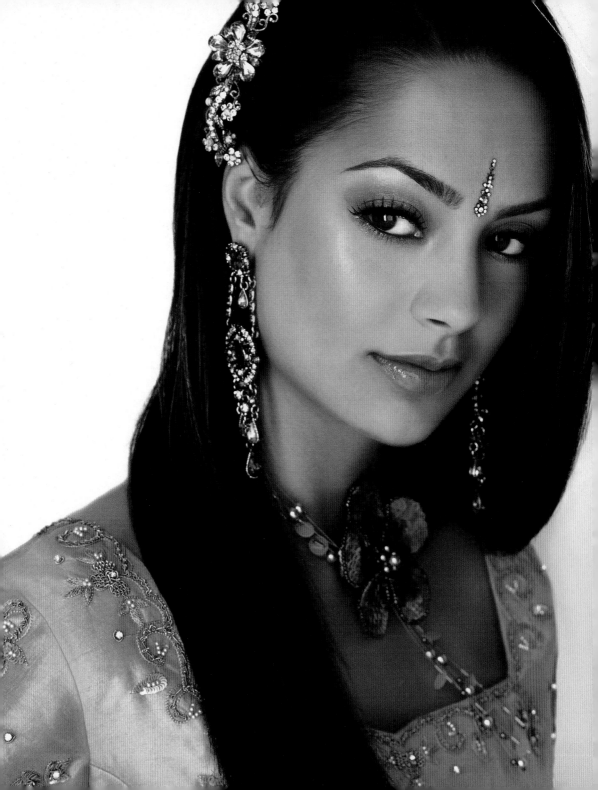

purple

THE LOOK
Make-up: Naveeda
Outfit: Rang Collection
Accessories: Rang Accessories
Bindis: Bombay Looks

MAKE-UP
Foundation: Mac Hypo Real foundation 600
Eyes: Mac eyeliner & mascara in Black, Elizabeth Arden Berry 11, Nars eye shadow Tibet, Vincent Longo Trio eye shadow Purple Sky
Cheeks: Iman Luxury Blushing Powder Peace
Lips: Stila Lip Glaze

HAIR
Products: Paul Mitchell Freeze and Shine Super Spray

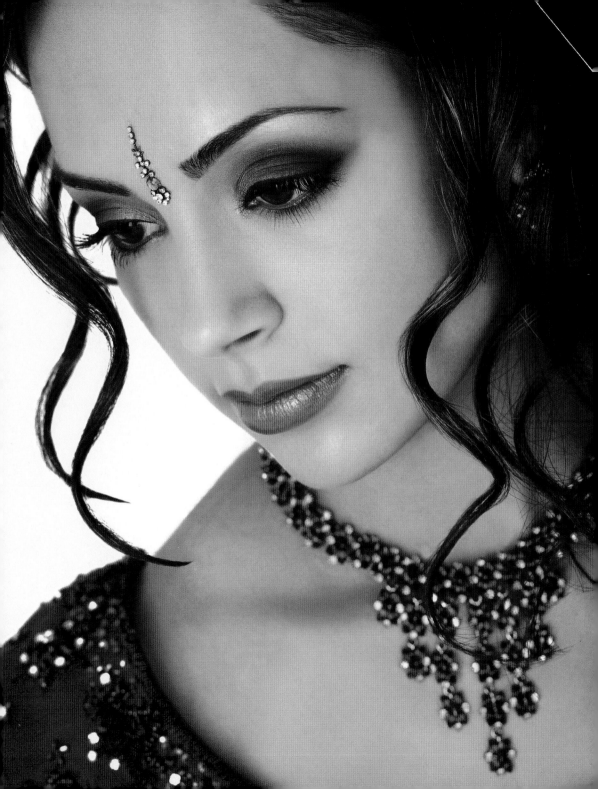

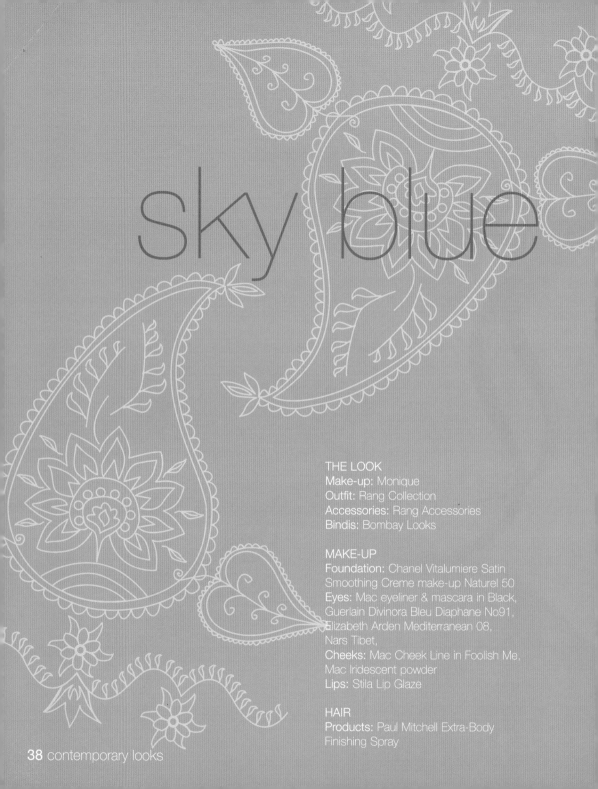

sky blue

THE LOOK
Make-up: Monique
Outfit: Rang Collection
Accessories: Rang Accessories
Bindis: Bombay Looks

MAKE-UP
Foundation: Chanel Vitalumiere Satin
Smoothing Creme make-up Naturel 50
Eyes: Mac eyeliner & mascara in Black,
Guerlain Divinora Bleu Diaphane No91,
Elizabeth Arden Mediterranean 08,
Nars Tibet,
Cheeks: Mac Cheek Line in Foolish Me,
Mac Iridescent powder
Lips: Stila Lip Glaze

HAIR
Products: Paul Mitchell Extra-Body
Finishing Spray

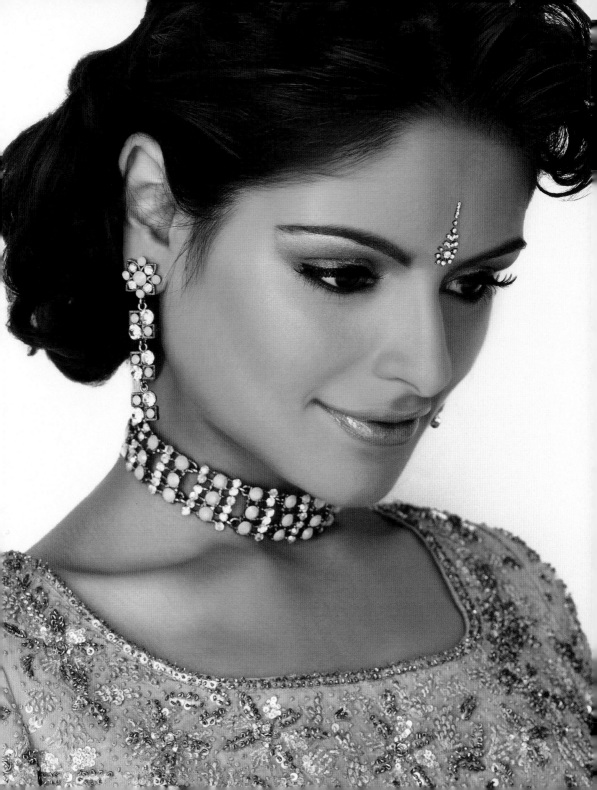

baby blue

THE LOOK
Make-up: Monique
Outfit: Trendz
Accessories: Rang Accessories

MAKE-UP
Foundation: Chanel Vitalumiere Satin Smoothing Creme make up Naturel 50
Eyes: Mac eyeliner & mascara in Black, RMK Mix Colors for Eyes Shiny Green 01, Guerlain Divinora Bleu Diaphane No.91, Nars Tibet,
Cheeks: Mac Cheek Line in Foolish Me, Mac Iridescent powder
Lips: Stila Lip Glaze

HAIR
Products: Paul Mitchell Freeze and Shine Super Spray

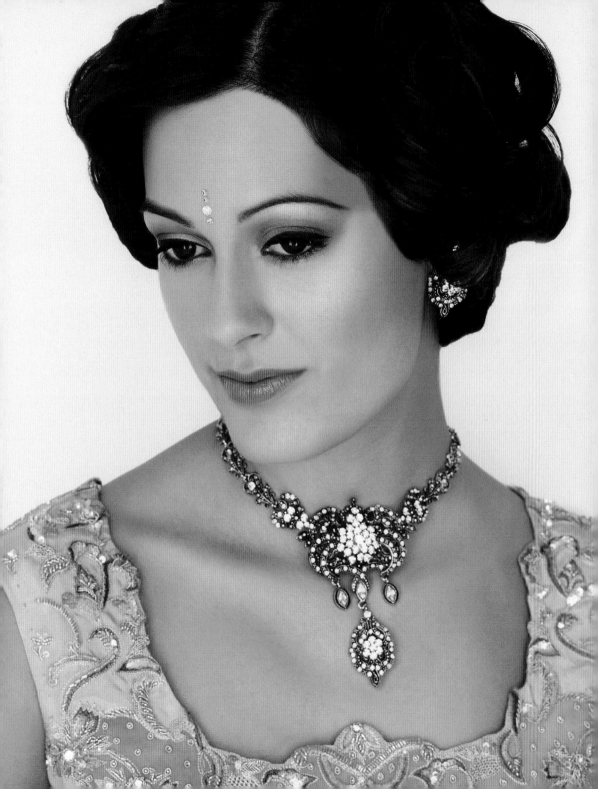

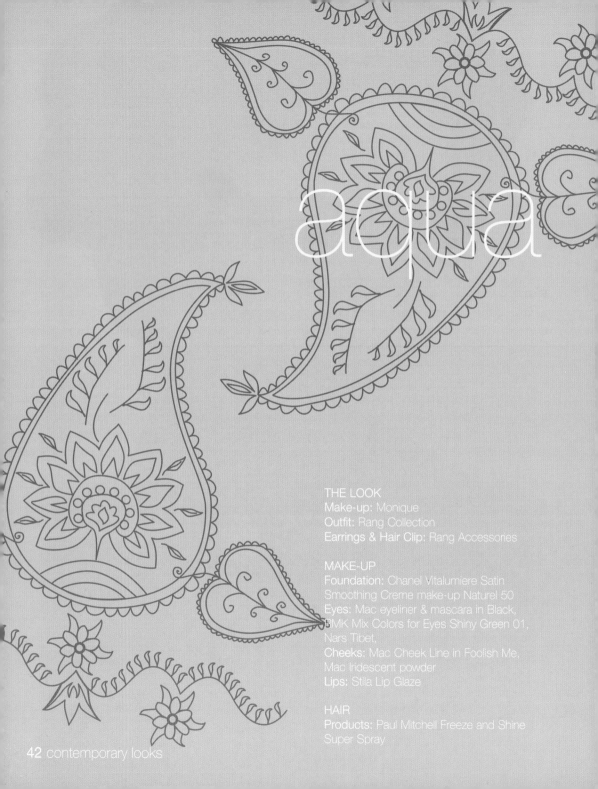

aqua

THE LOOK
Make-up: Monique
Outfit: Rang Collection
Earrings & Hair Clip: Rang Accessories

MAKE-UP
Foundation: Chanel Vitalumiere Satin
Smoothing Creme make-up Naturel 50
Eyes: Mac eyeliner & mascara in Black,
BMK Mix Colors for Eyes Shiny Green 01,
Nars Tibet,
Cheeks: Mac Cheek Line in Foolish Me,
Mac Iridescent powder
Lips: Stila Lip Glaze

HAIR
Products: Paul Mitchell Freeze and Shine
Super Spray

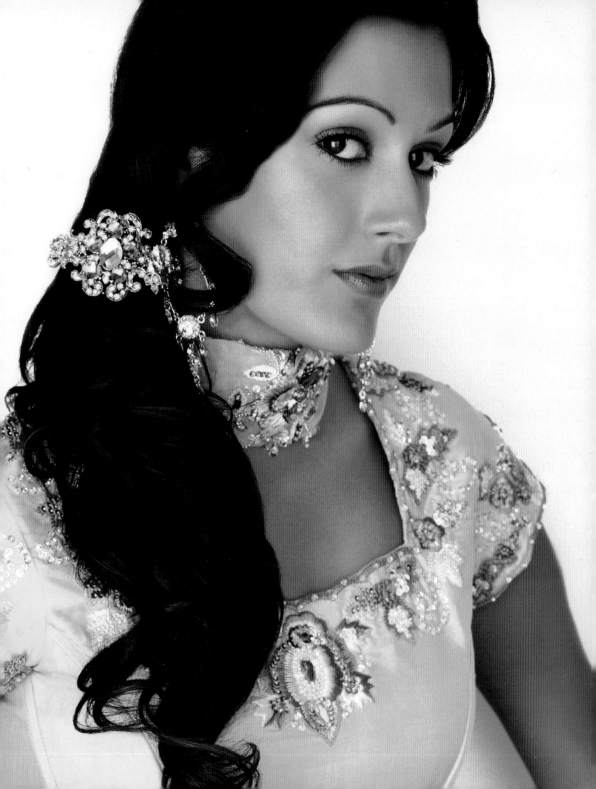

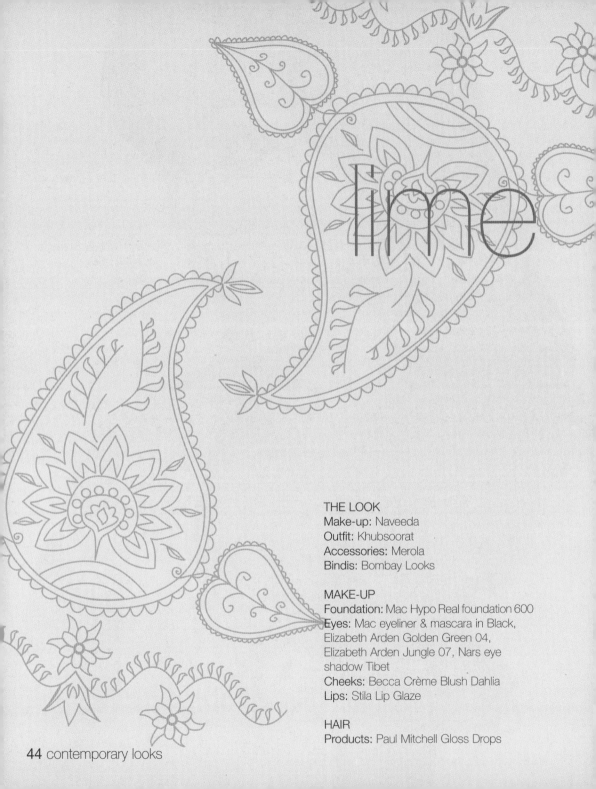

lime

THE LOOK
Make-up: Naveeda
Outfit: Khubsoorat
Accessories: Merola
Bindis: Bombay Looks

MAKE-UP
Foundation: Mac Hypo Real foundation 600
Eyes: Mac eyeliner & mascara in Black,
Elizabeth Arden Golden Green 04,
Elizabeth Arden Jungle 07, Nars eye
shadow Tibet
Cheeks: Becca Crème Blush Dahlia
Lips: Stila Lip Glaze

HAIR
Products: Paul Mitchell Gloss Drops

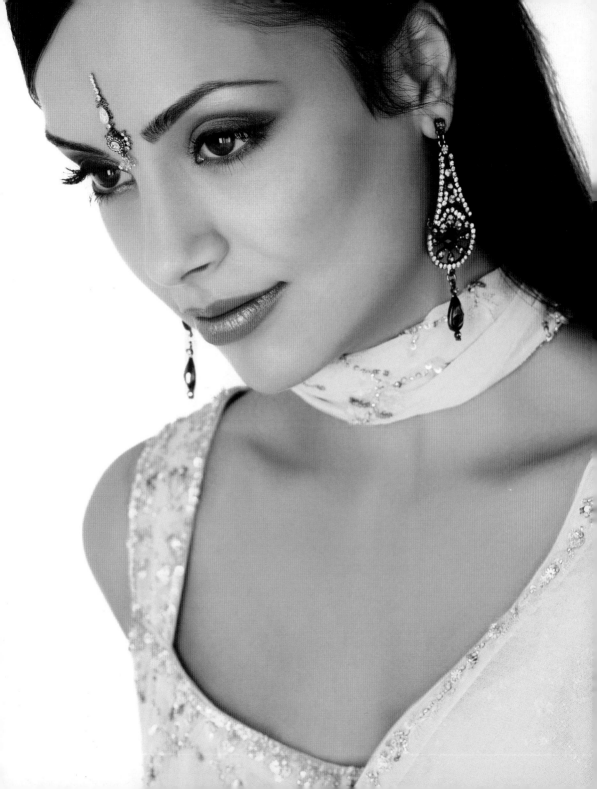

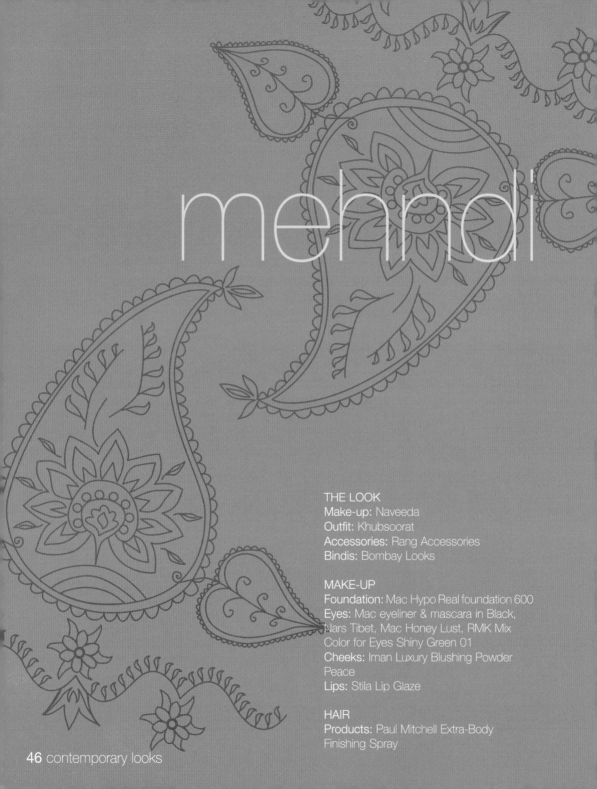

mehndi

THE LOOK
Make-up: Naveeda
Outfit: Khubsoorat
Accessories: Rang Accessories
Bindis: Bombay Looks

MAKE-UP
Foundation: Mac Hypo Real foundation 600
Eyes: Mac eyeliner & mascara in Black,
Nars Tibet, Mac Honey Lust, RMK Mix
Color for Eyes Shiny Green 01
Cheeks: Iman Luxury Blushing Powder
Peace
Lips: Stila Lip Glaze

HAIR
Products: Paul Mitchell Extra-Body
Finishing Spray

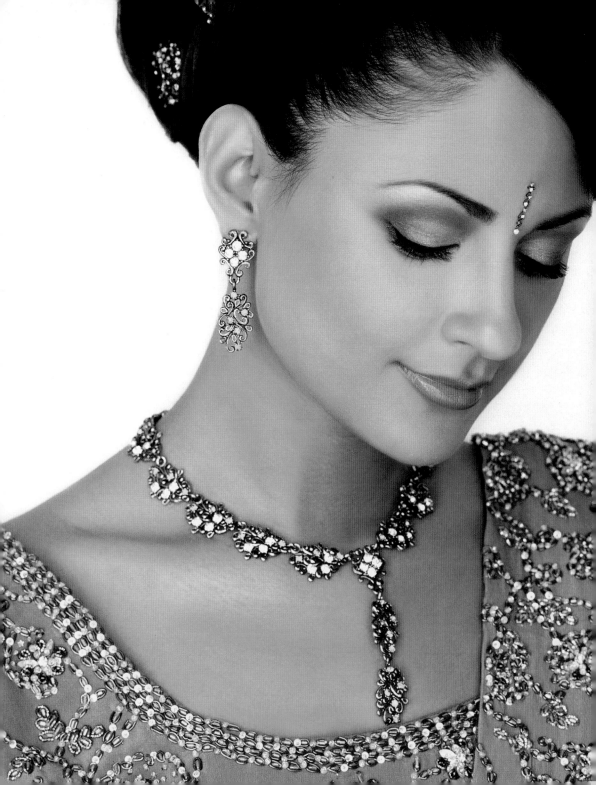

gold dust

THE LOOK
Make-up: Nina Haider
Outfit: Rang Collection
Accessories: Rang Accessories

MAKE-UP
Foundation: Becca Luminous Skin Colour Nut
Eyes: Lancome Color Focus 108 Casque D'or, Mac-Honey Lust, Mac eyeliner in Black, Clinique High Impact mascara Black/Brown 02, Ruby & Millie Eye Color Yellow 210P
Cheeks: Becca Creme Blush Dahlia, Ruby & Millie Face & Body Metal Gold
Lips: Mac Satin Spirit A93, Becca Glossy Lip Tint Frisco

HAIR
Products: Paul Mitchell Extra-Body Finishing Spray

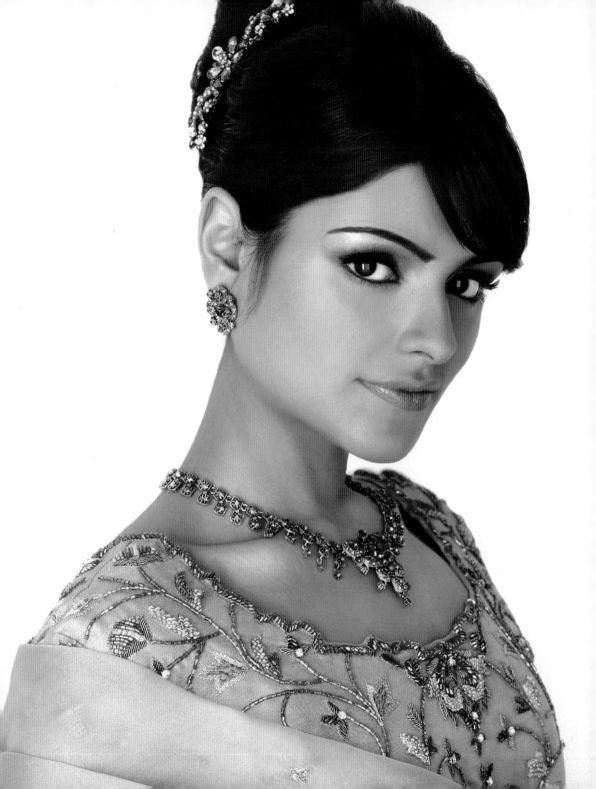

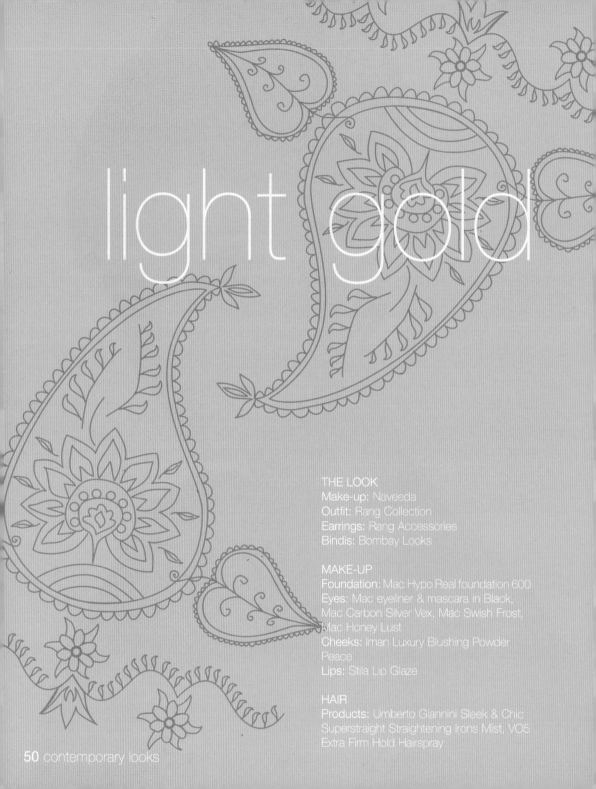

light gold

THE LOOK
Make-up: Naveeda
Outfit: Rang Collection
Earrings: Rang Accessories
Bindis: Bombay Looks

MAKE-UP
Foundation: Mac Hypo Real foundation 600
Eyes: Mac eyeliner & mascara in Black,
Mac Carbon Silver Vex, Mac Swish Frost,
Mac Honey Lust
Cheeks: Iman Luxury Blushing Powder
Peace
Lips: Stila Lip Glaze

HAIR
Products: Umberto Giannini Sleek & Chic
Superstraight Straightening Irons Mist, VO5
Extra Firm Hold Hairspray

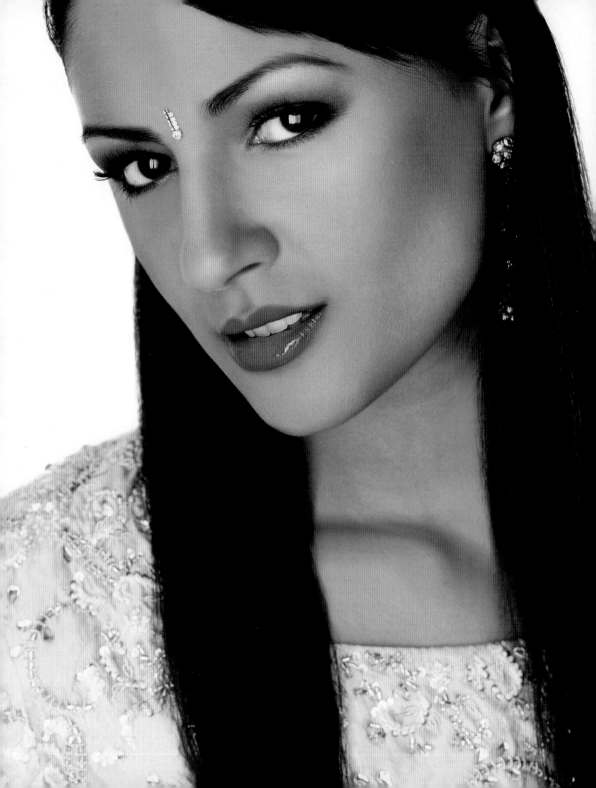

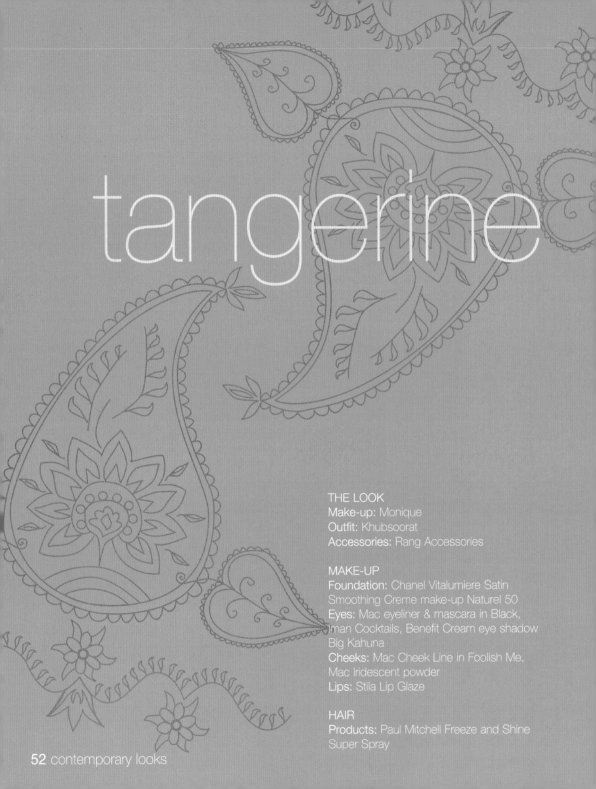

tangerine

THE LOOK
Make-up: Monique
Outfit: Khubsoorat
Accessories: Rang Accessories

MAKE-UP
Foundation: Chanel Vitalumiere Satin
Smoothing Creme make-up Naturel 50
Eyes: Mac eyeliner & mascara in Black,
Iman Cocktails, Benefit Cream eye shadow
Big Kahuna
Cheeks: Mac Cheek Line in Foolish Me,
Mac Iridescent powder
Lips: Stila Lip Glaze

HAIR
Products: Paul Mitchell Freeze and Shine
Super Spray

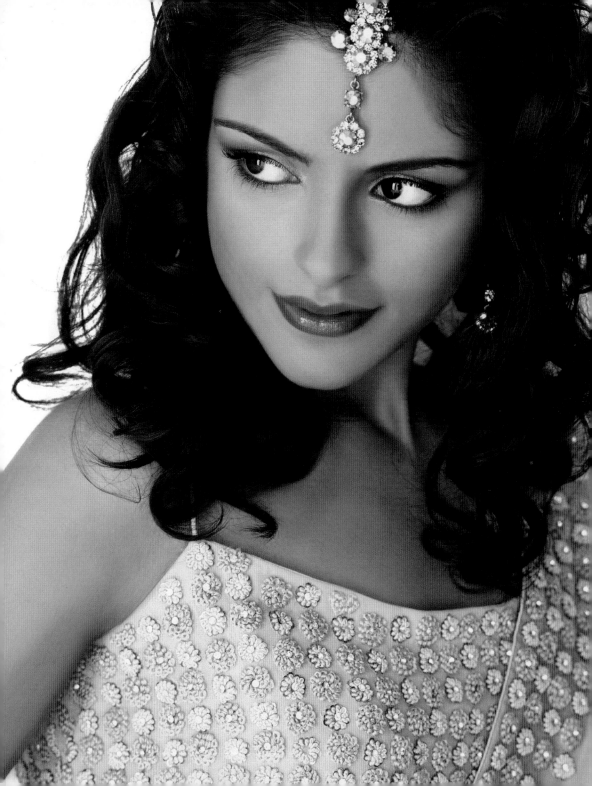

burnt orange

THE LOOK
Make-up: Naveeda
Outfit: Bombay Looks
Earrings & Earring used as a tikka: Rang Accessories
Bindis: Bombay Looks

MAKE-UP
Foundation: Mac Hypo Real foundation 600
Eyes: Mac eyeliner & mascara in Black, Elizabeth Arden Mediterranean 08, Elizabeth Arden Pumpkin 02, Nars eye shadow Tibet, Benefit Cream eye shadow Big Kahuna
Cheeks: Becca Crème Blush Dahlia
Lips: Mac Satin Spirit A93, Becca Glossy Lip Tint Frisco, Nars Velvet Matte lip pencil Forbidden Red

HAIR
Products: Paul Mitchell Extra Body Finishing Spray

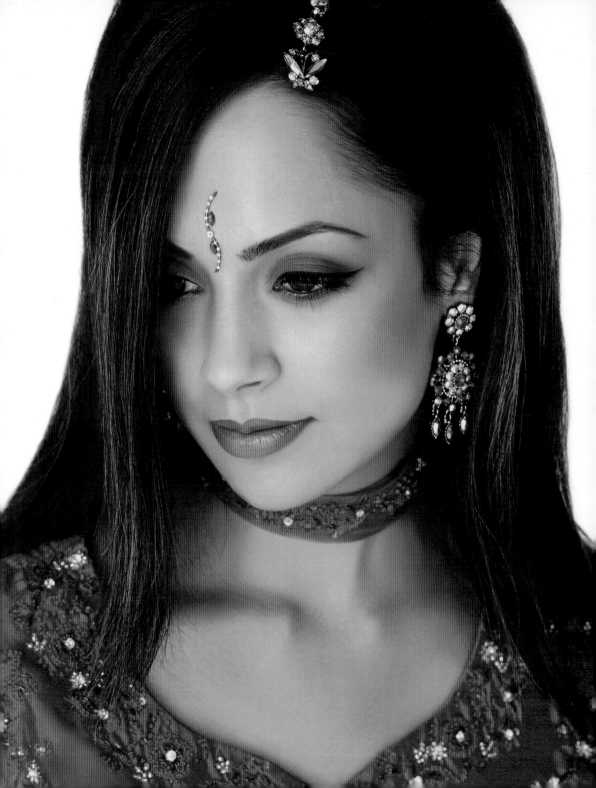

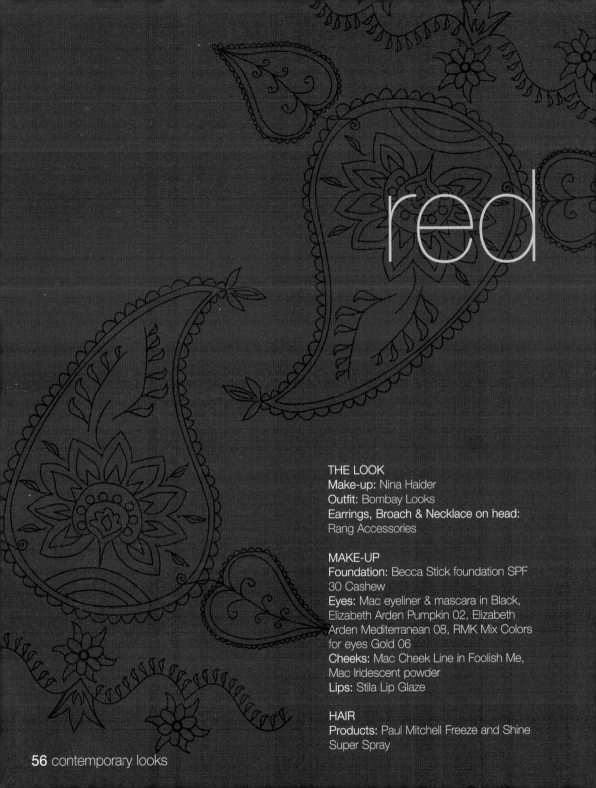

red

THE LOOK
Make-up: Nina Haider
Outfit: Bombay Looks
Earrings, Broach & Necklace on head:
Rang Accessories

MAKE-UP
Foundation: Becca Stick foundation SPF
30 Cashew
Eyes: Mac eyeliner & mascara in Black,
Elizabeth Arden Pumpkin 02, Elizabeth
Arden Mediterranean 08, RMK Mix Colors
for eyes Gold 06
Cheeks: Mac Cheek Line in Foolish Me,
Mac Iridescent powder
Lips: Stila Lip Glaze

HAIR
Products: Paul Mitchell Freeze and Shine
Super Spray

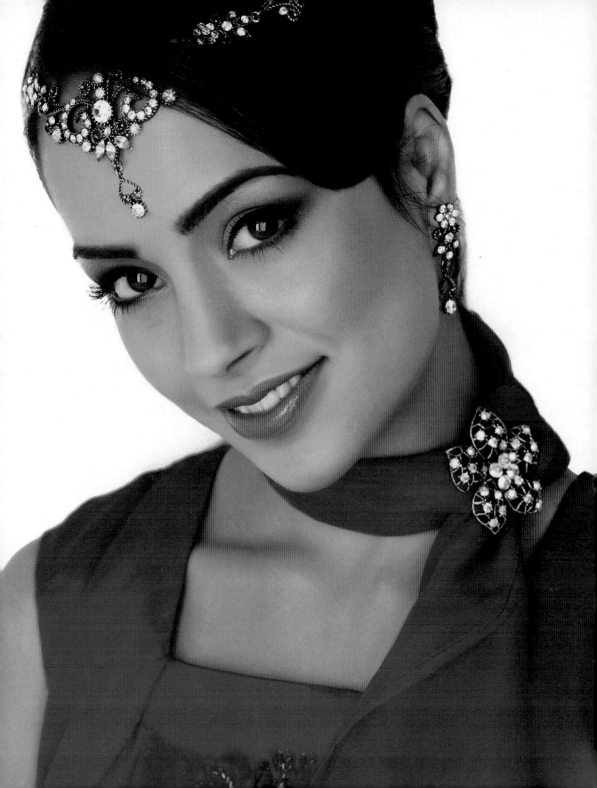

maroon

THE LOOK
Make-up: Monique
Outfit: Trendz
Earrings & Tiara: Bombay Looks

MAKE-UP
Foundation: Chanel Double Perfection
(crème powder make-up)
Eyes: Mac eye liner & mascara in Black,
Lancôme Color Focus eye shadow
Casque D'or 108, Mac Honey Lust,
Nars Tibet
Cheeks: Mac Cheek Line in Foolish Me,
Mac Iridescent powder
Lips: Stila Lip Glaze

HAIR
Products: Vo5 Extra Firm Hold Hairspray,
Paul Mitchell The Shine Instant Spray-on-
Shine

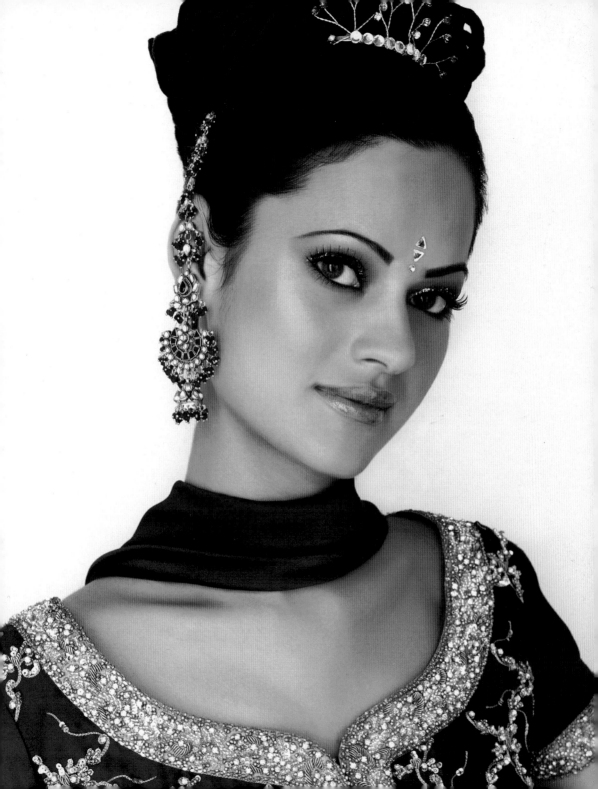

plum

THE LOOK
Make-up: Nina Haider
Outfit: Rang Collection
Accessories: Rang Accessories
Tiara & Bindi: Bombay Looks

MAKE-UP
Foundation: Becca Luminous Skin Colour
Nut D2
Eyes: Mac eyeliner & mascara in Black,
Elizabeth Arden Petal Pink 10, Iman
Rendezvous
Cheeks: Mac Cheek Line in Foolish Me,
Mac Iridescent powder
Lips: Iman Luxury Lip Shimmer Velvet

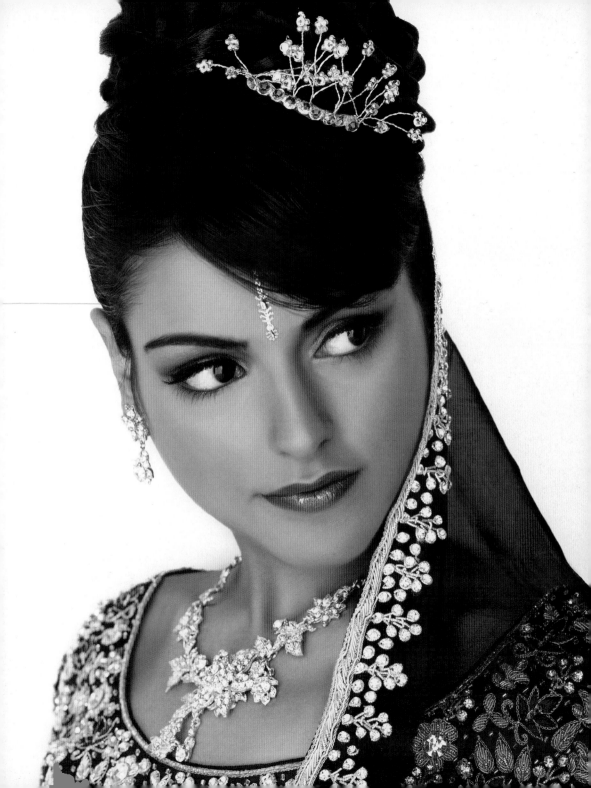

hot pink

THE LOOK
Make-up: Monique
Outfit: Trendz
Accessories: Rang Accessories

MAKE-UP
Foundation: Chanel Double Perfection
(crème powder make-up)
Eyes: Mac eye liner & mascara in Black,
Nars Tibet, Elizabeth Arden Berry 11
Cheeks: Mac Cheek Line in Foolish Me,
Mac Iridescent powder
Lips: Stila Lip Glaze

HAIR
Products: Vo5 Extra Firm Hold Hairspray,
Paul Mitchell The Shine Instant Spray-on-
Shine

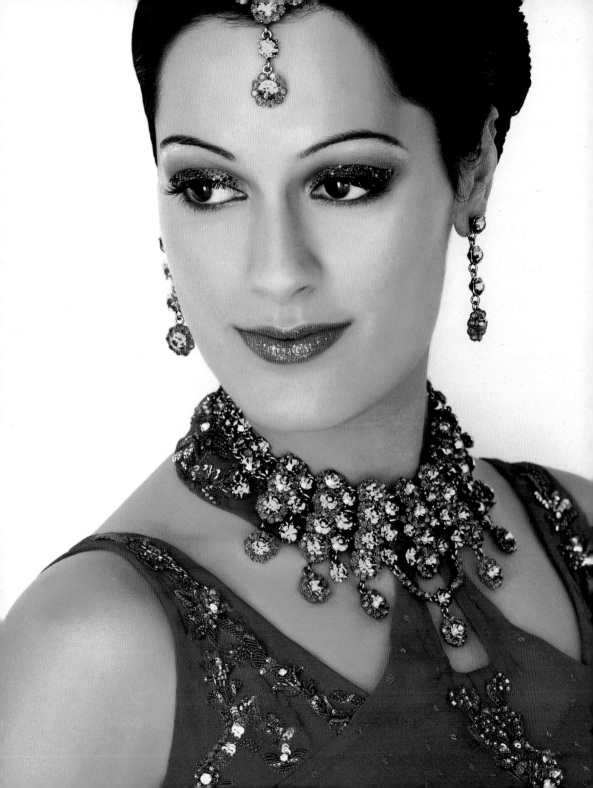

salmon & red

THE LOOK
Make-up: Naveeda
Outfit: Trendz
Accessories: Rang Accessories
Bindis: Bombay Looks

MAKE-UP
Foundation: Mac Hypo Real foundation 600
Eyes: Mac eyeliner & mascara in Black, Benefit cream eye shadow Big Kahuna, Mac Honey Lust, Elizabeth Arden Pumpkin 02
Cheeks: Iman Luxury Blushing Powder Peace
Lips: Clinique Plush Red 13, Nars Velvet Matte lip pencil Forbidden Red

HAIR
Products: Paul Mitchell Extra-Body Finishing Spray

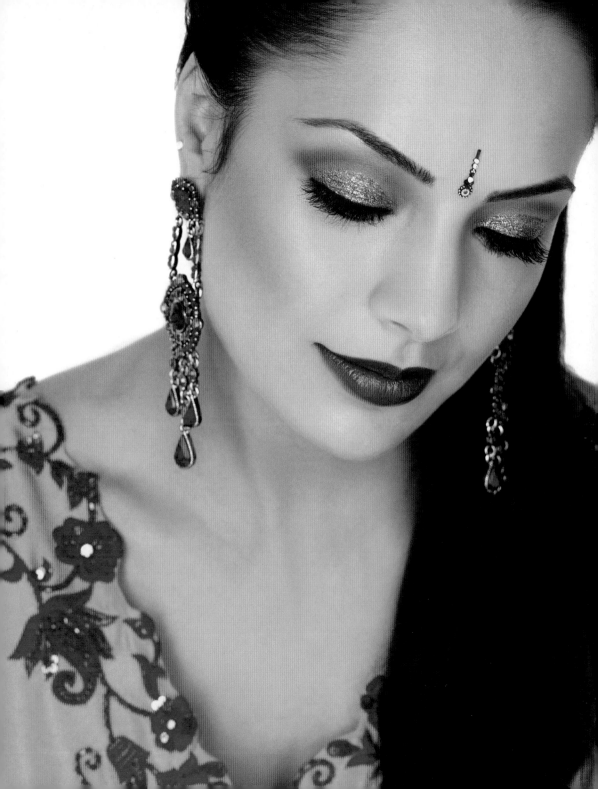

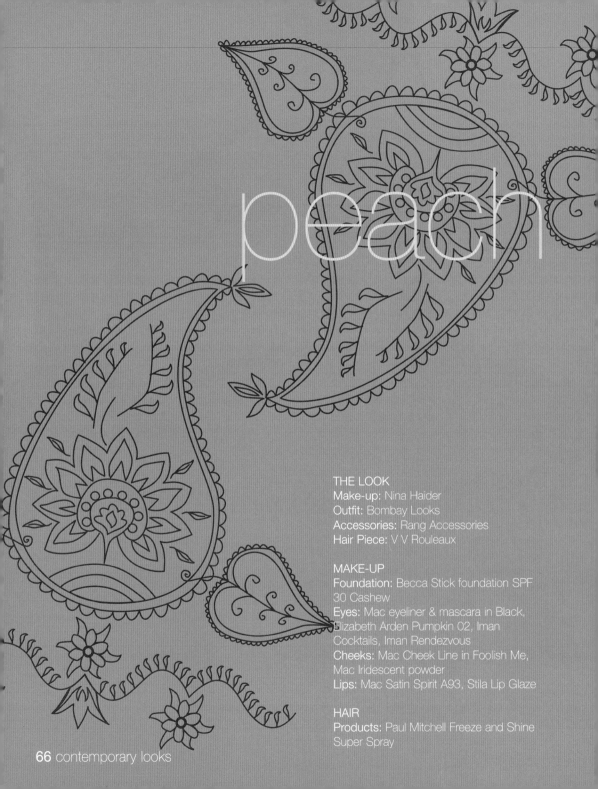

peach

THE LOOK
Make-up: Nina Haider
Outfit: Bombay Looks
Accessories: Rang Accessories
Hair Piece: V V Rouleaux

MAKE-UP
Foundation: Becca Stick foundation SPF 30 Cashew
Eyes: Mac eyeliner & mascara in Black, Elizabeth Arden Pumpkin 02, Iman Cocktails, Iman Rendezvous
Cheeks: Mac Cheek Line in Foolish Me, Mac Iridescent powder
Lips: Mac Satin Spirit A93, Stila Lip Glaze

HAIR
Products: Paul Mitchell Freeze and Shine Super Spray

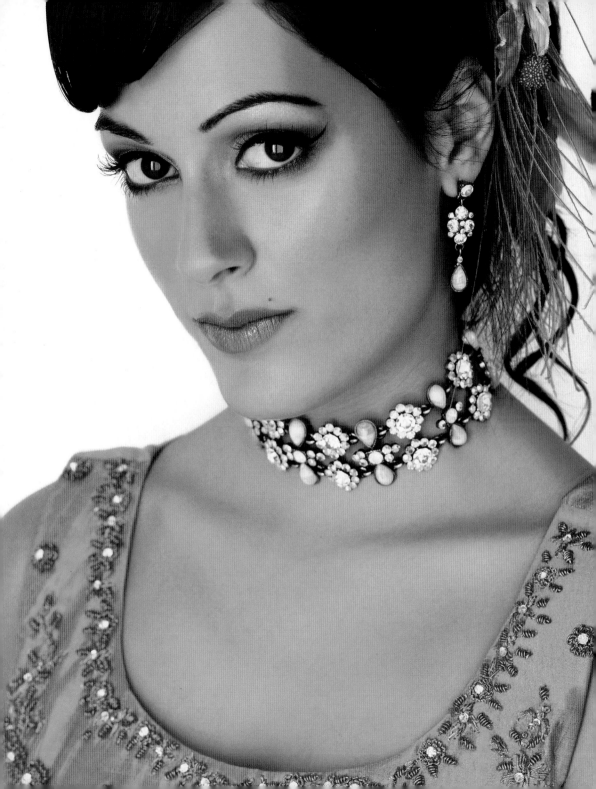

peach &
turquoise

THE LOOK
Make-up: Nina Haider
Outfit: Khubsoorat
Accessories: Rang Accessories

MAKE-UP
Foundation: Becca Stick foundation SPF 30 Cashew
Eyes: Mac eyeliner & mascara in Black. Elizabeth Arden Pumpkin 02, Elizabeth Arden Mediterranean 08, Benefit Cream eye shadow Big Kahuna
Cheeks: Mac Cheek Line in Foolish Me. Mac Iridescent powder
Lips: Stila Lip Glaze

HAIR
Products: Paul Mitchell Extra-Body Finishing Spray

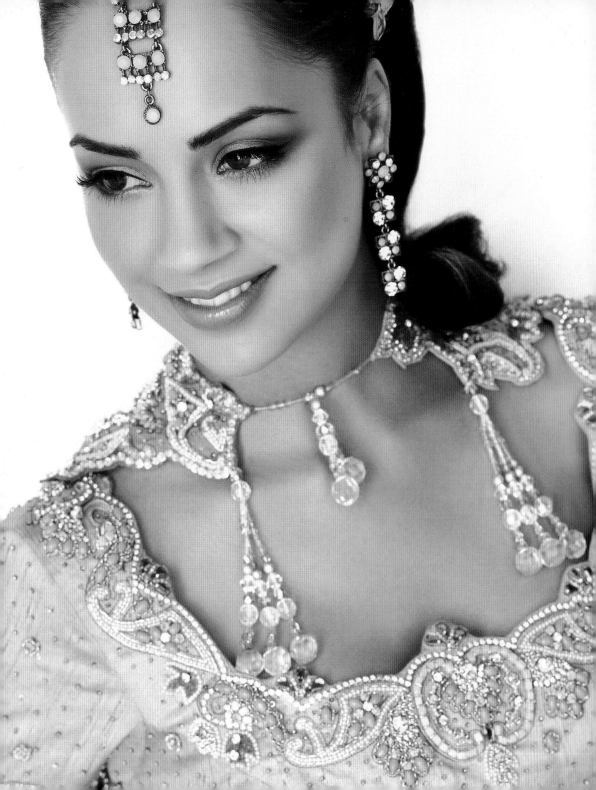

Chapter 2

classic looks

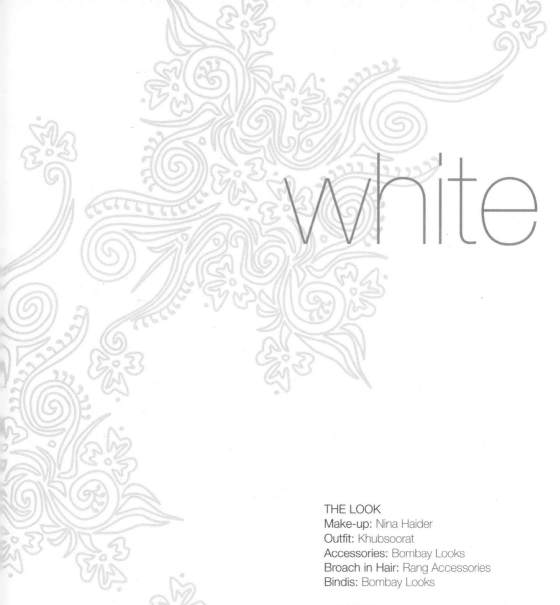

white

THE LOOK
Make-up: Nina Haider
Outfit: Khubsoorat
Accessories: Bombay Looks
Broach in Hair: Rang Accessories
Bindis: Bombay Looks

MAKE-UP
Foundation: Becca Stick foundation SPF
30 Cashew
Eyes: Mac eyeliner & mascara in Black,
Nars eye shadow Tibet, Bobbi Brown
Shimmer Wash eye shadow Sterling 12
Cheeks: Mac Cheek Line in Foolish Me,
Mac Iridescent powder
Lips: Stila Lip Glaze

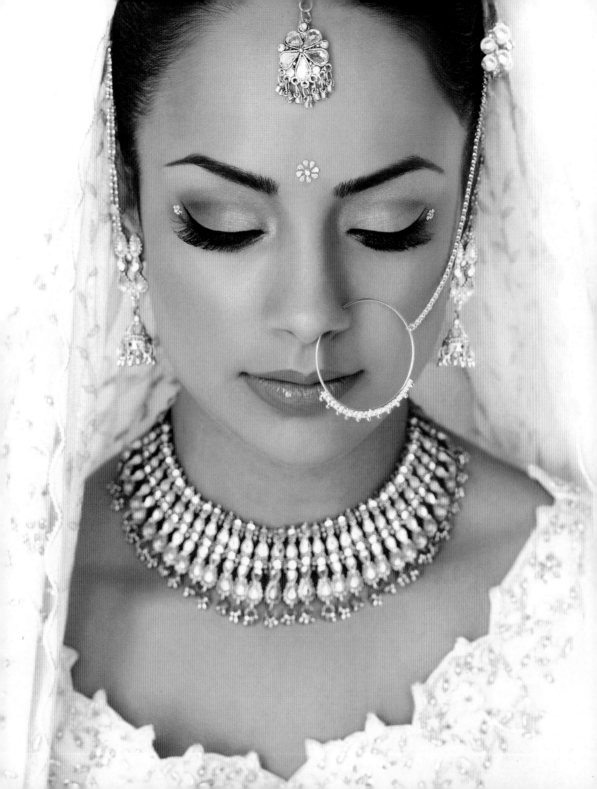

off white

THE LOOK
Make-up: Naveeda
Outfit: Payal Collection
Necklace: Merola
Earrings, Tikka & Bindi: Bombay Looks

MAKE-UP
Foundation: Mac Hypo Real foundation 600
Powder: Mac Studio Fix C4
Eyes: Lancome Color Focus 108 Casque
D'or, Mac Honey Lust, Stila eyes cheek &
lip palette, Mac eyeliner in Black, Clinique
High Impact mascara Black/Brown 02
Cheeks: Prescriptives Powder
Cheekcolor Refillable
Lips: Revlon Cappuccino, Stila Lip Glaze

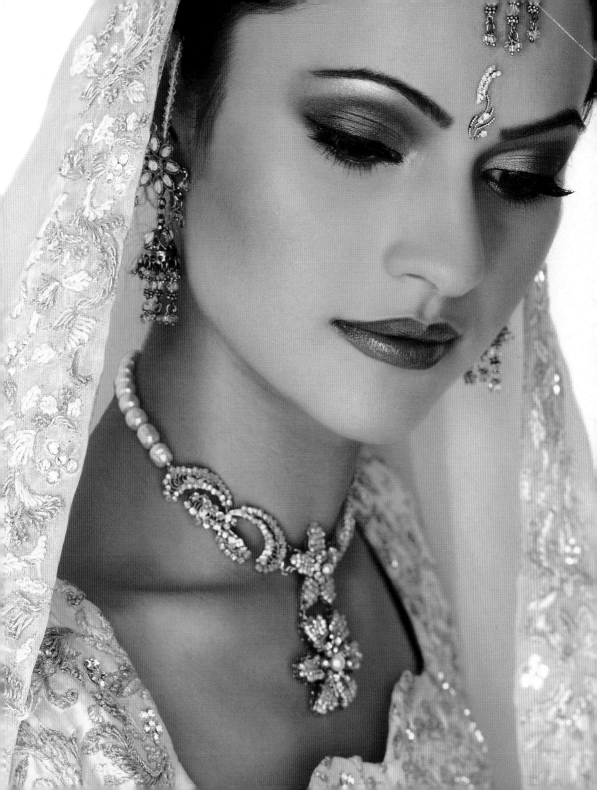

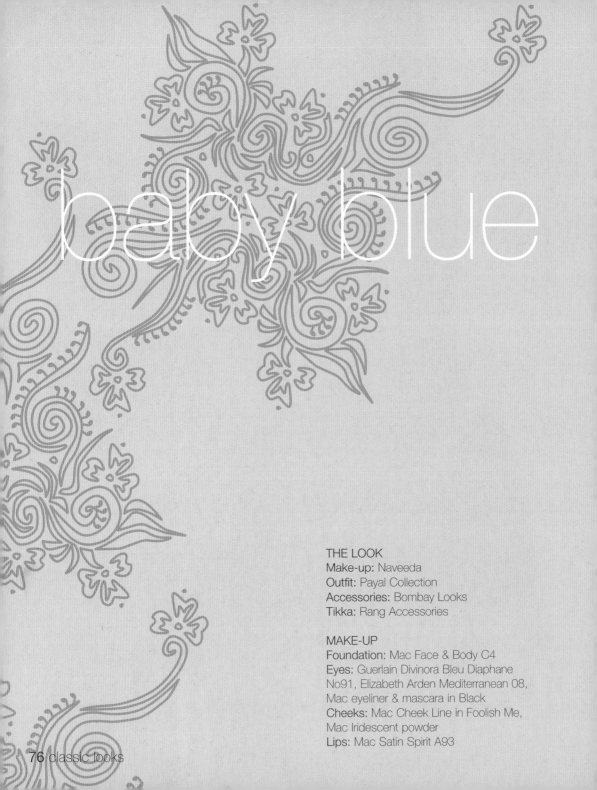

baby blue

THE LOOK
Make-up: Naveeda
Outfit: Payal Collection
Accessories: Bombay Looks
Tikka: Rang Accessories

MAKE-UP
Foundation: Mac Face & Body C4
Eyes: Guerlain Divinora Bleu Diaphane
No91, Elizabeth Arden Mediterranean 08,
Mac eyeliner & mascara in Black
Cheeks: Mac Cheek Line in Foolish Me,
Mac Iridescent powder
Lips: Mac Satin Spirit A93

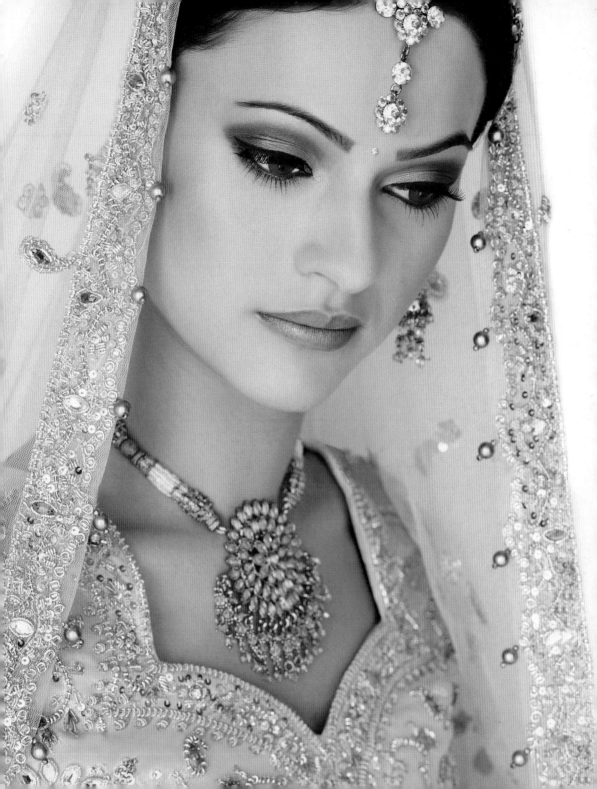

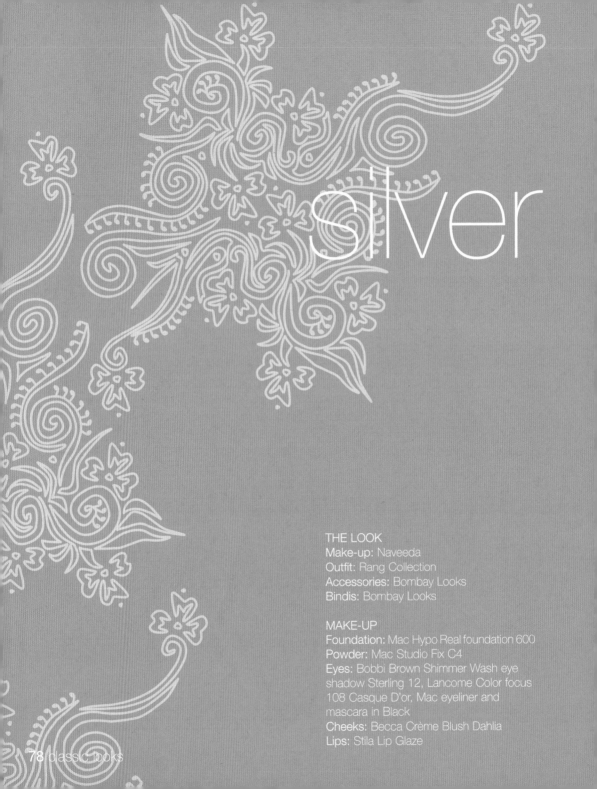

silver

THE LOOK
Make-up: Naveeda
Outfit: Rang Collection
Accessories: Bombay Looks
Bindis: Bombay Looks

MAKE-UP
Foundation: Mac Hypo Real foundation 600
Powder: Mac Studio Fix C4
Eyes: Bobbi Brown Shimmer Wash eye shadow Sterling 12, Lancome Color focus 108 Casque D'or, Mac eyeliner and mascara in Black
Cheeks: Becca Crème Blush Dahlia
Lips: Stila Lip Glaze

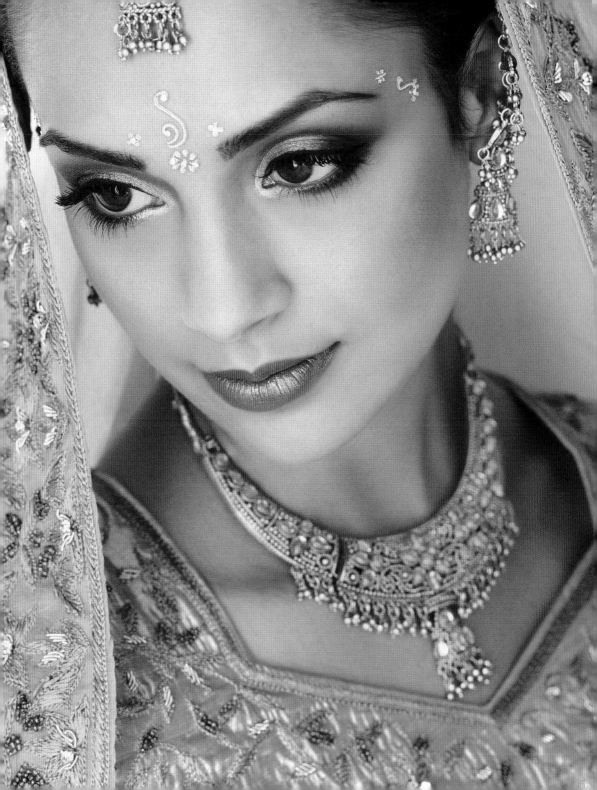

lilac

THE LOOK
Make-up: Naveeda
Outfit: Rang Collection
Accessories: Rang Accessories

MAKE-UP
Foundation: Mac Face & Body C4
Eyes: Iman Rendezvous, Elizabeth Arden
Petal Pink, Mac eyeliner in Black, Clinique
High Impact mascara Black/Brown 02
Cheeks: Mac Cheek Line in Foolish Me,
Mac Iridescent powder
Lips: Stila Lip Glaze

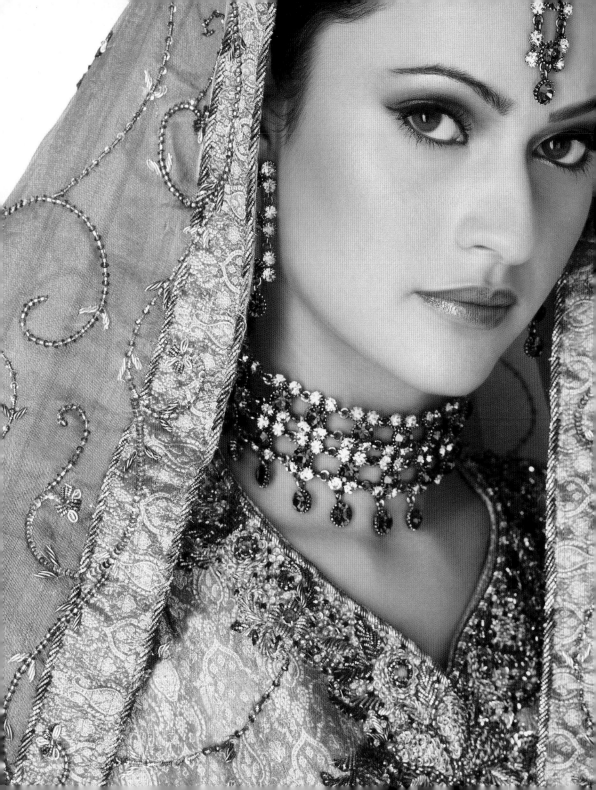

baby pink

THE LOOK
Make-up: Nina Haider
Outfit: Payal Collection
Accessories: Bombay Looks
Bindis: Bombay Looks

MAKE-UP
Foundation: Becca Stick foundation SPF 30 Cashew
Eyes: Mac eyeliner & mascara in Black, Elizabeth Arden Petal Pink 10, Elizabeth Arden Mediterranean 08, Nars eye shadow Tibet, Iman Cocktails
Cheeks: Mac Cheek Line in Foolish Me, Mac Iridescent powder
Lips: Stila Lip Glaze

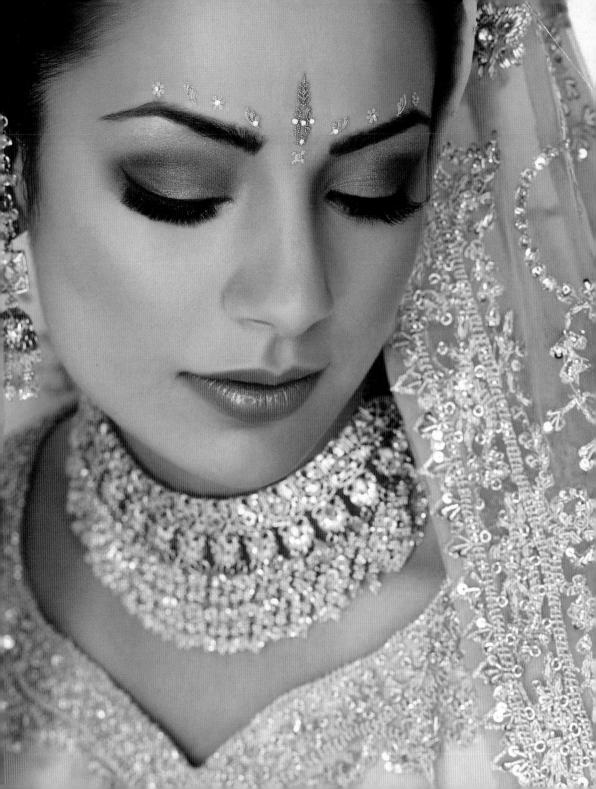

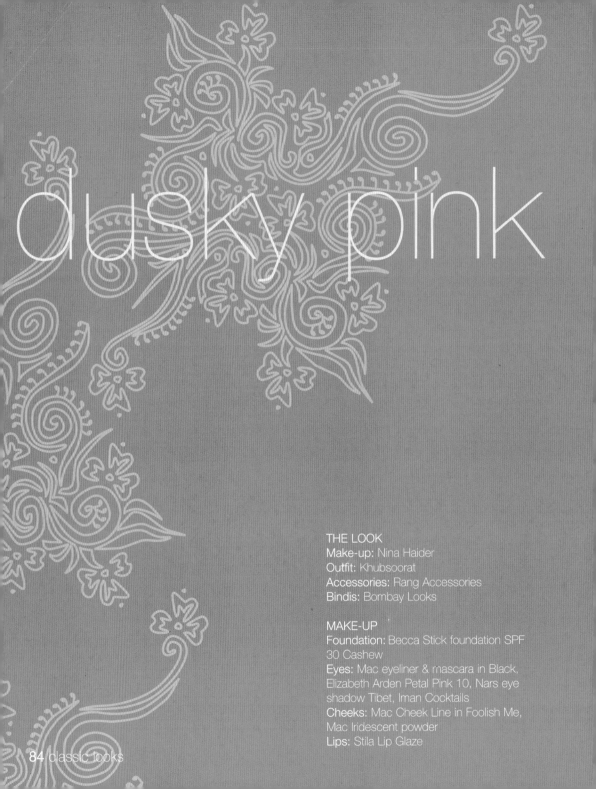

dusky pink

THE LOOK
Make-up: Nina Haider
Outfit: Khubsoorat
Accessories: Rang Accessories
Bindis: Bombay Looks

MAKE-UP
Foundation: Becca Stick foundation SPF 30 Cashew
Eyes: Mac eyeliner & mascara in Black, Elizabeth Arden Petal Pink 10, Nars eye shadow Tibet, Iman Cocktails
Cheeks: Mac Cheek Line in Foolish Me, Mac Iridescent powder
Lips: Stila Lip Glaze

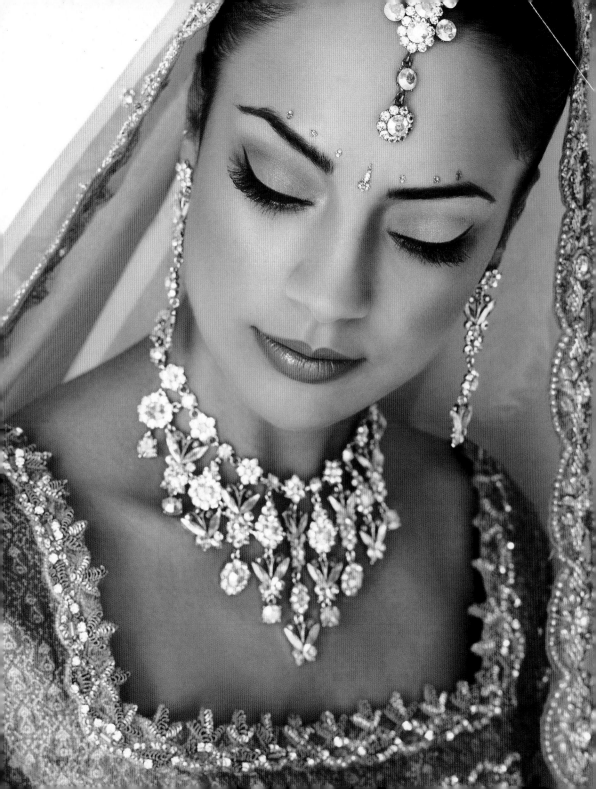

hot pink

THE LOOK
Make-up: Naveeda
Outfit: Khubsoorat
Accessories: Bombay Looks
Tikka: Rang Accessories
Bindis: Bombay Looks

MAKE-UP
Foundation: Mac Hypo Real foundation 600
Mac Studio Fix powder C4
Eyes: Mac eyeliner & mascara in Black,
Givenchy eye shadow Fuchsia 04,
Iman Cocktails
Cheeks: Mac Cream Colour Base
Flamming Fuchsia
Lips: Guerlain Divinora No260, Nars Velvet
Matte Lip Pencil Damned

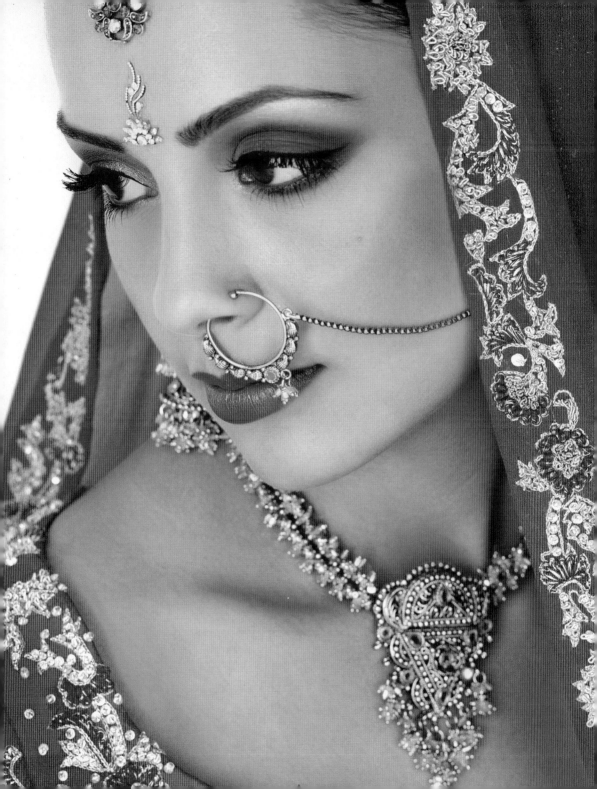

burnt orange

THE LOOK
Make-up: Nina Haider
Outfit: Payal Collection
Accessories: Rang Accessories
Bindis: Bombay Looks

MAKE-UP
Foundation: Becca Stick foundation SPF 30 Cashew
Eyes: Mac eyeliner & mascara in Black, Benefit cream eye shadow Big Kahuna, Nars eye shadow Tibet, Mac Honey Lust
Cheeks: Mac Cheek Line in Foolish Me, Mac Iridescent powder
Lips: Mac lipstick Satin Spirit A93, Becca Glossy Lip Tint Frisco

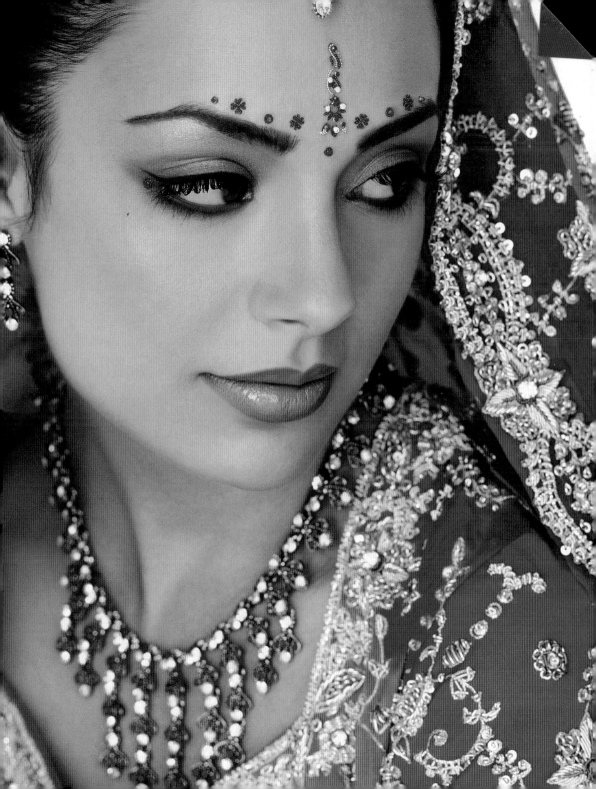

cherry red & diamante

THE LOOK
Make-up: Nina Haider
Outfit: Khubsoorat
Accessories: Rang Accessories
Bindis: Bombay Looks

MAKE-UP
Foundation: Becca Stick foundation SPF 30 Cashew
Eyes: Mac eyeliner & mascara in Black, Mac Pigment Colour Powder Vanilla A83
Cheeks: Mac Cream Colour Base Flamming Fuchsia
Lips: Clinique Plush Red 13, Nars Velvet Matte lip pencil Forbidden Red

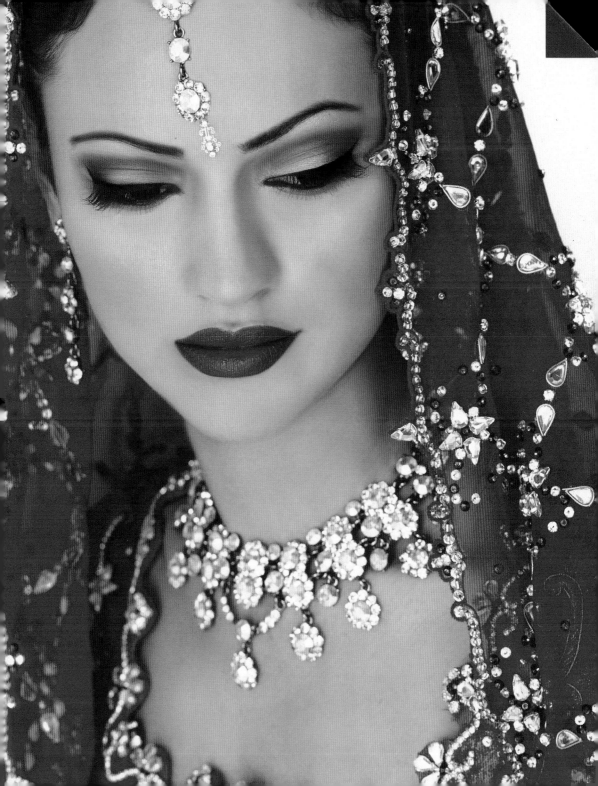

crimson

THE LOOK
Make-up: Naveeda
Outfit: Payal Collection
Accessories: Bombay Looks
Bindis: Bombay Looks

MAKE-UP
Foundation: Mac Hypo Real foundation 600
Eyes: Mac eyeliner & mascara in Black,
Mac Honey Lust, RMK Mix Color for eyes
Gold 06
Cheeks: Becca Crème Blush Dahlia
Lips: Elizabeth Arden Colour Intrigue
lipstick Dare 02

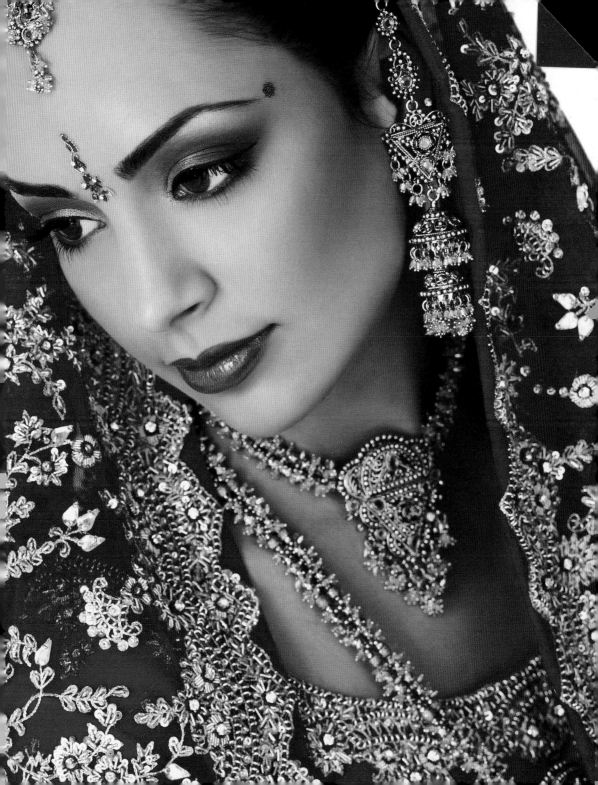

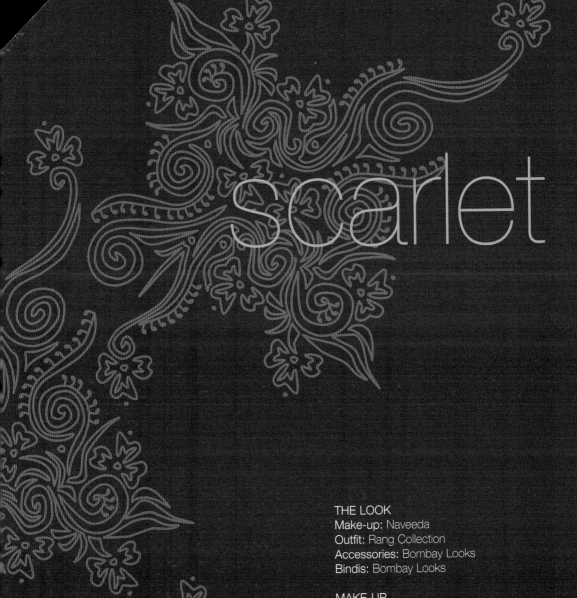

scarlet

THE LOOK
Make-up: Naveeda
Outfit: Rang Collection
Accessories: Bombay Looks
Bindis: Bombay Looks

MAKE-UP
Foundation: Mac Face & Body C4
Eyes: Lancome Color Focus 108 Casque
D'or Mac-Honey Lust, Mac eyeliner in
Black, Clinique High Impact mascara
Black/Brown 02
Cheeks: Mac Cheek Line in Foolish Me,
Mac Iridescent powder
Lips: Nars Velvet matte lip pencil Damned,
Stila Lip Glaze

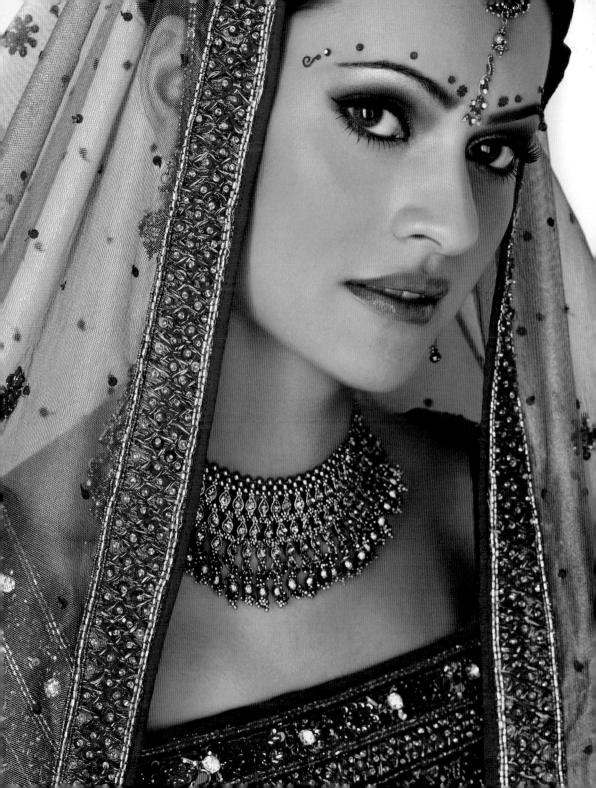

maroon

THE LOOK
Make-up: Nina Haider
Outfit: Payal Collection
Accessories: Bombay Looks
Bindis: Bombay Looks

MAKE-UP
Foundation: Becca Stick foundation SPF 30 Cashew
Eyes: Mac eyeliner & mascara in Black, Mac Honey Lust, Mac Pigment Colour powder Vanilla
Cheeks: Mac Cheek Line in Foolish Me, Mac Iridescent powder
Lips: Nars Velvet matte lip pencil Damned, Kiehl's Light lip gloss Golden Berry

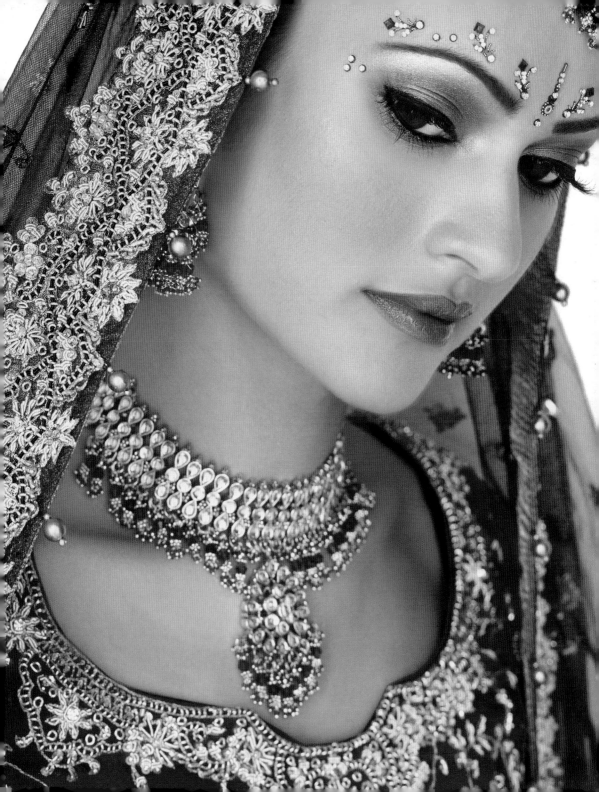

burgundy
& diamante

THE LOOK
Make-up: Naveeda
Outfit: Khubsoorat
Accessories: Rang Accessories
Bindis: Bombay Looks

MAKE-UP
Foundation: Mac Hypo Real foundation 600
Eyes: Mac eyeliner & mascara in Black, Nars eye shadow Tibet, Elizabeth Arden Berry 11, Mac Honey Lust
Cheeks: Iman Luxury Blushing Powder Peace
Lips: Elizabeth Arden Colour Intrigue lipstick Drama 04, Nars Velvet Matte lip pencil Damned

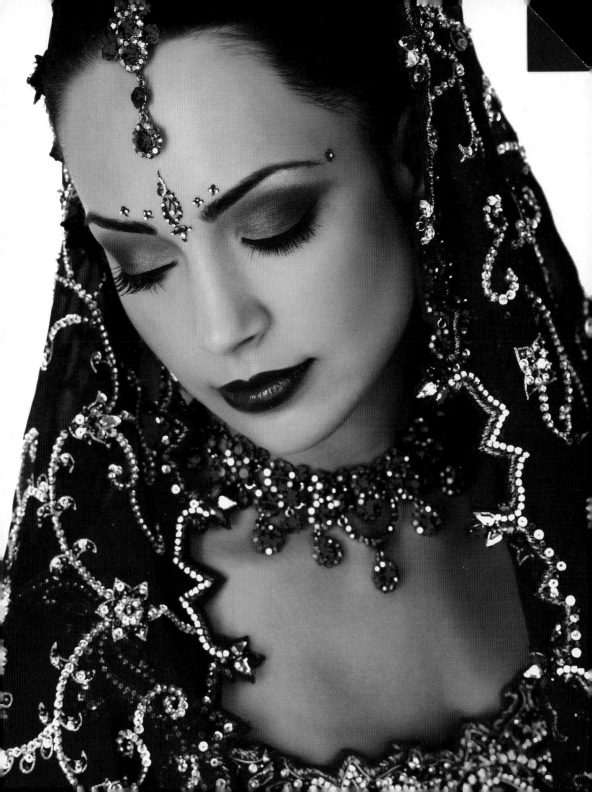

antique
burgundy

THE LOOK
Make-up: Nina Haider
Outfit: Payal Collection
Accessories: Bombay Looks
Bindis: Bombay Looks

MAKE-UP
Foundation: Mac Face & Body C4
Eyes: Nars Tibet, Mac Honey Lust, Mac
eyeliner and mascara in Black,
Iman Rendezvous
Cheeks: Mac Cheek Line in Foolish Me,
Mac Iridescent powder
Lips: Mac Satin Spirit A93, Becca Glossy
Lip Tint Frisco

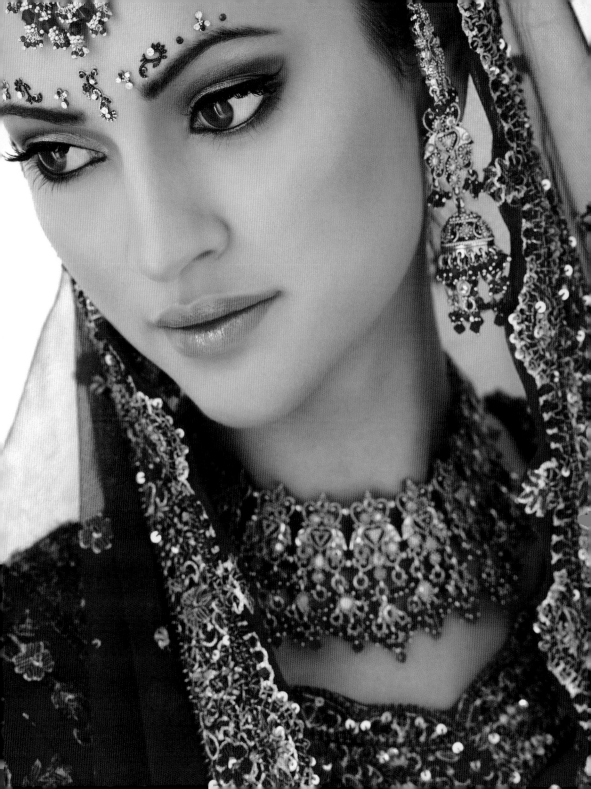

brown

THE LOOK
Make-up: Naveeda
Outfit: Payal Collection
Accessories: Bombay Looks
Bindis: Bombay Looks

MAKE-UP
Foundation: Becca Stick foundation SPF
30 Cashew
Eyes: Mac eyeliner & mascara in Black,
Lancôme Color Focus eye shadow
Casque D'or 108, RMK Mix Colors for
eyes Gold 06, Nars eye shadow Tibet
Cheeks: Mac Cheek Line in Foolish Me,
Mac Iridescent powder
Lips: Iman Luxury Moisturising Lipstick,
Iman Luxury Lip Shimmer Velvet

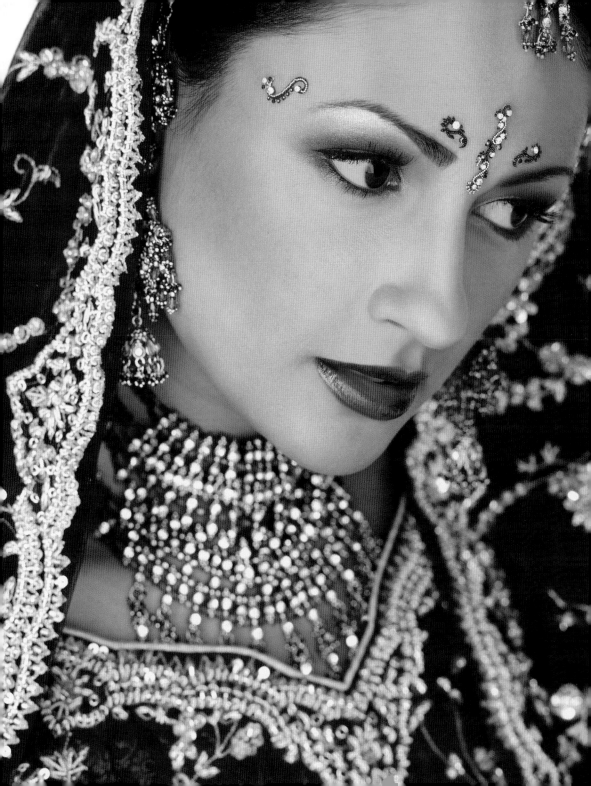

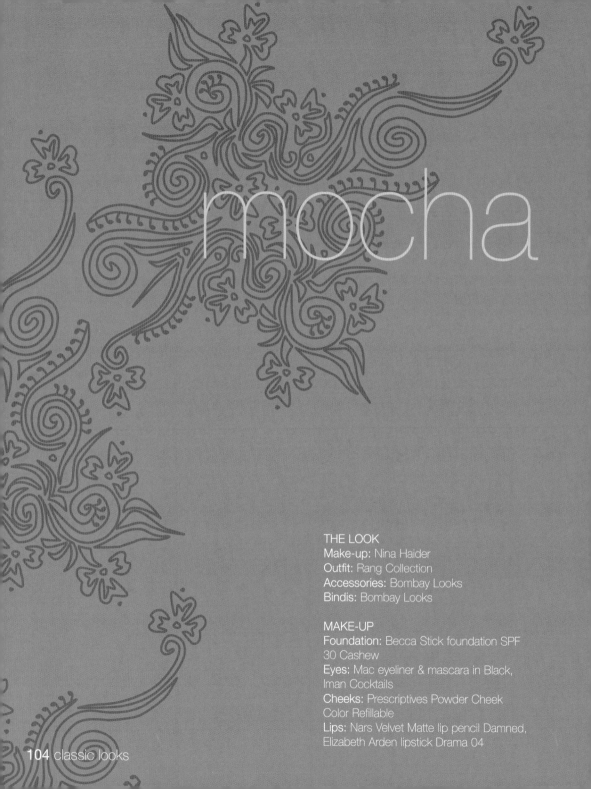

mocha

THE LOOK
Make-up: Nina Haider
Outfit: Rang Collection
Accessories: Bombay Looks
Bindis: Bombay Looks

MAKE-UP
Foundation: Becca Stick foundation SPF 30 Cashew
Eyes: Mac eyeliner & mascara in Black, Iman Cocktails
Cheeks: Prescriptives Powder Cheek Color Refillable
Lips: Nars Velvet Matte lip pencil Damned, Elizabeth Arden lipstick Drama 04

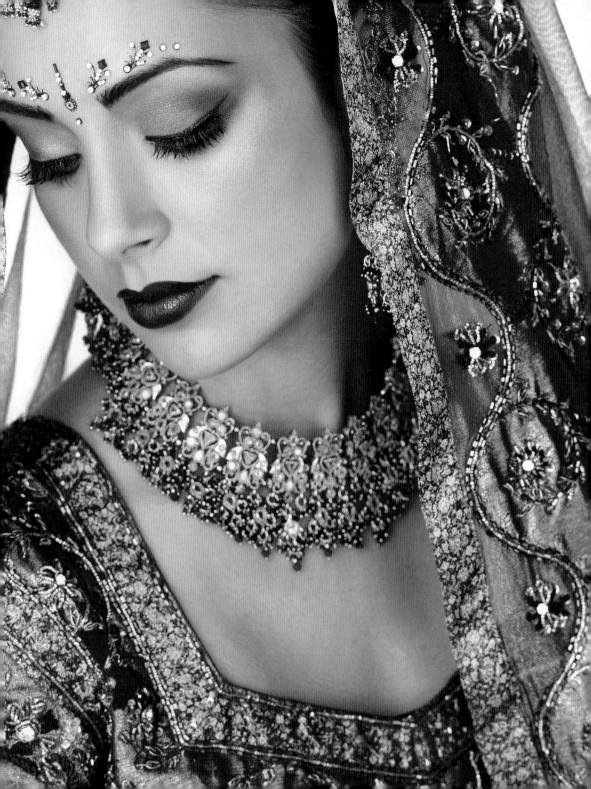

mehndi

THE LOOK

THE LOOK
Make-up: Nina Haider
Outfit: Trendz
Accessories: Bombay Looks
Bindis: Bombay Looks

MAKE-UP
Foundation: Mac Face & Body C4
Eyes: Mac eyeliner & mascara in Black,
Elizabeth Arden Jungle 07, RMK Mix
Colors for Eyes Gold 06, Iman
Rendezvous
Cheeks: Mac Cheek Line in Foolish Me,
Mac Iridescent powder
Lips: Stila Lip Glaze

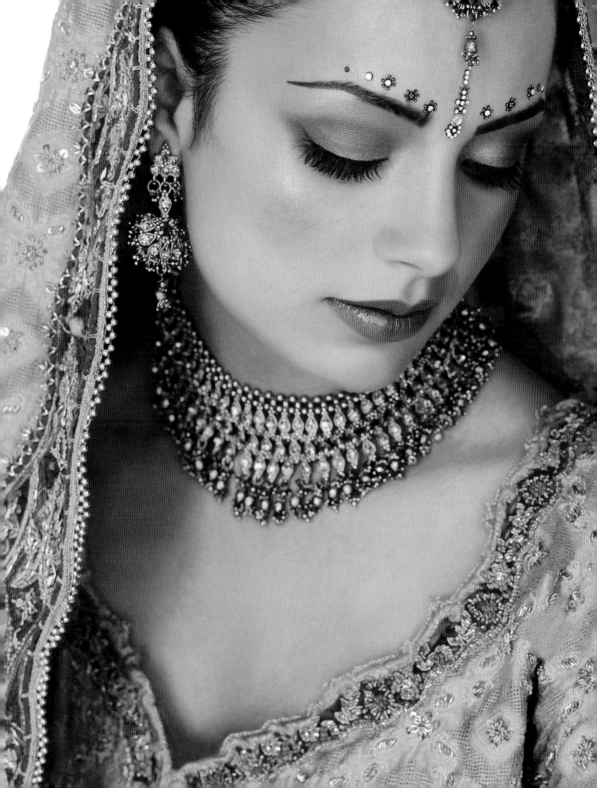

champagne gold

THE LOOK
Make-up: Naveeda
Outfit: Rang Collection
Accessories: Bombay Looks
Bindis: Bombay Looks

MAKE-UP
Foundation: Mac Hypo Real foundation 600
Powder: Mac Studio Fix C4
Eyes: Lancome Color Focus 108 Casque d'or, Iman Cocktails, Elizabeth Arden Eyeliner in black 01, Mac Mascara in Black
Cheeks: Prescriptives Powder Cheek Color Refillable
Lips: Revlon Cappuccino, Stila Lip Glaze

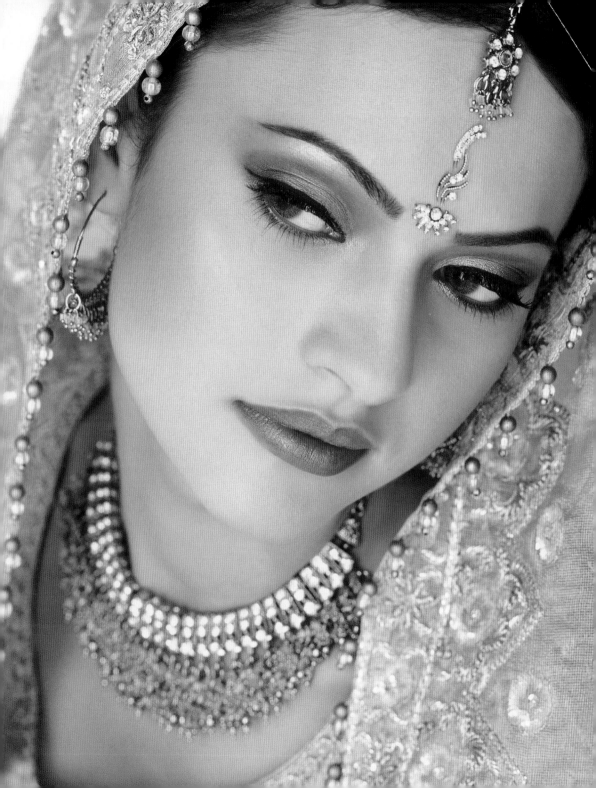

light gold

THE LOOK
Make-up: Nina Haider
Outfit: Payal Collection
Accessories: Bombay Looks
Bindis: Bombay Looks

MAKE-UP
Foundation: Becca Stick foundation SPF 30 Cashew
Eyes: Mac eyeliner & mascara in Black, Lancome Color Focus 108 Casque D'or Mac Pigment Colour Powder Vanilla, Elizabeth Arden Mediterranean 08
Cheeks: Mac Cheek Line in Foolish Me, Mac Iridescent powder
Lips: Nars Velvet Matte lip pencil Forbidden Red, Stila Lip Glaze

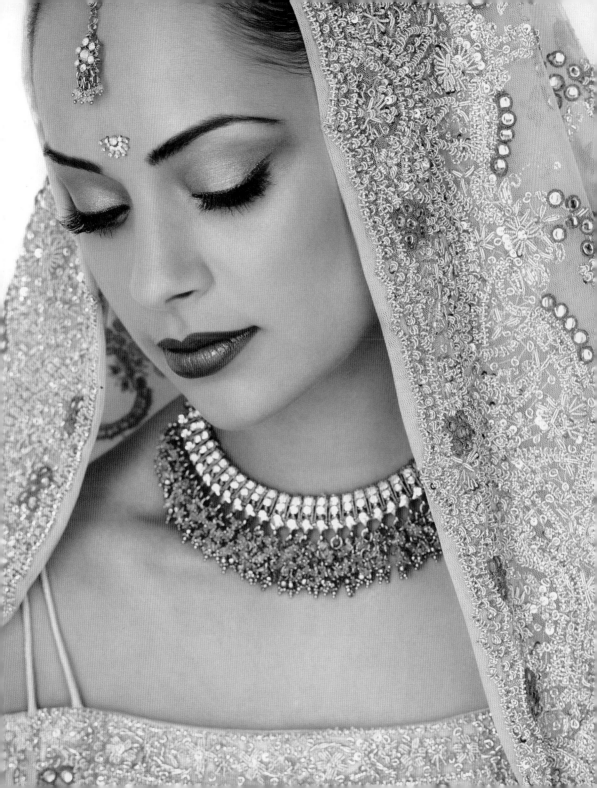

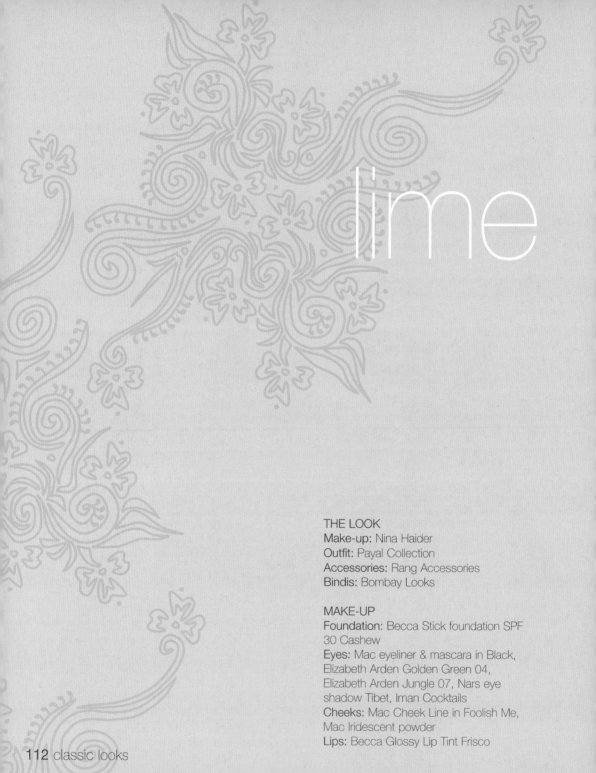

lime

THE LOOK
Make-up: Nina Haider
Outfit: Payal Collection
Accessories: Rang Accessories
Bindis: Bombay Looks

MAKE-UP
Foundation: Becca Stick foundation SPF 30 Cashew
Eyes: Mac eyeliner & mascara in Black, Elizabeth Arden Golden Green 04, Elizabeth Arden Jungle 07, Nars eye shadow Tibet, Iman Cocktails
Cheeks: Mac Cheek Line in Foolish Me, Mac Iridescent powder
Lips: Becca Glossy Lip Tint Frisco

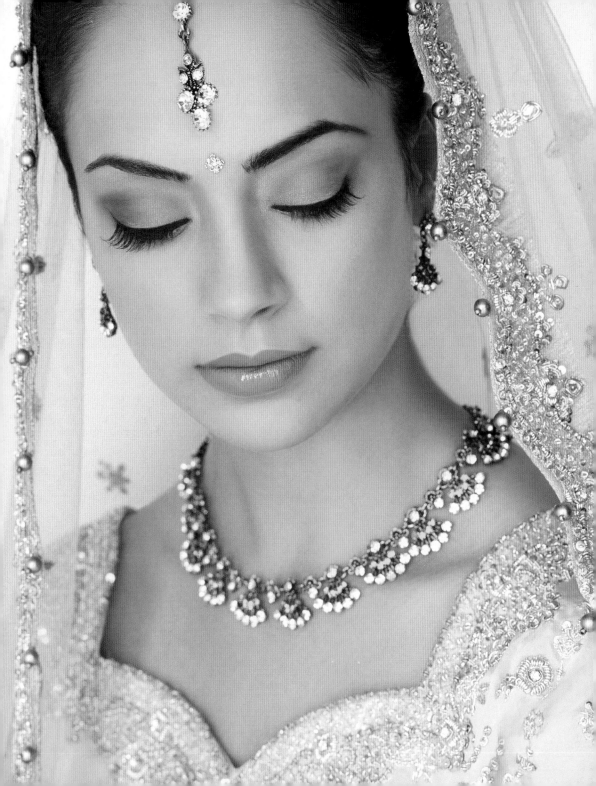

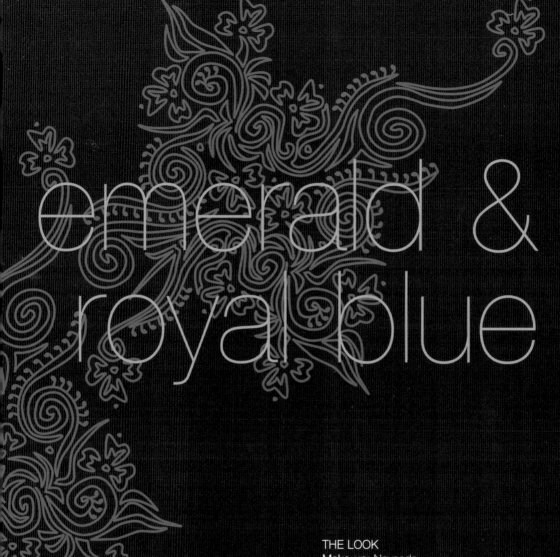

emerald &
royal blue

THE LOOK
Make-up: Naveeda
Outfit: Rang Collection
Accessories: Bombay Looks
Bindis: Bombay Looks

MAKE-UP
Foundation: Mac Face & Body C4
Eyes: Elizabeth Arden Mediterranean 08,
Elizabeth Arden Jungle 07,
Mac Black mascara
Cheeks: Prescriptives Powder Cheek
Color Refillable
Lips: Mac Satin Spirit A93

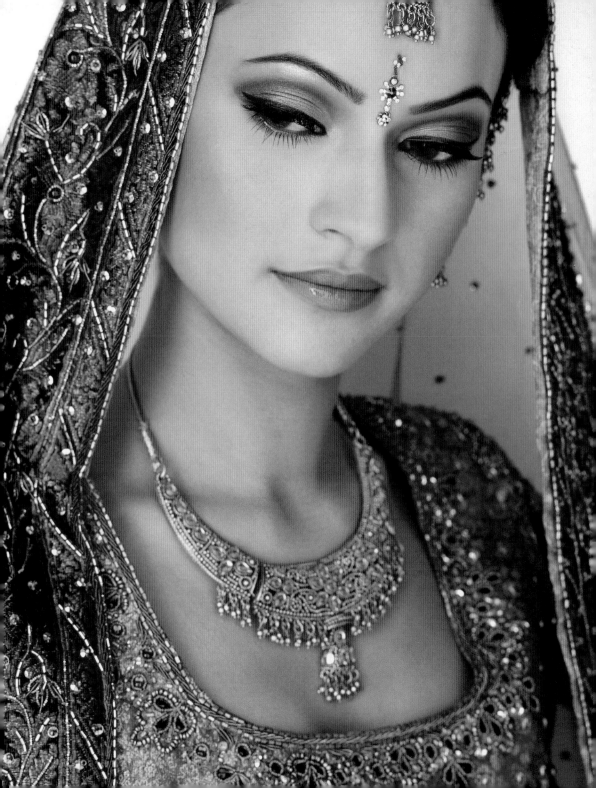

Chapter 3

hair looks

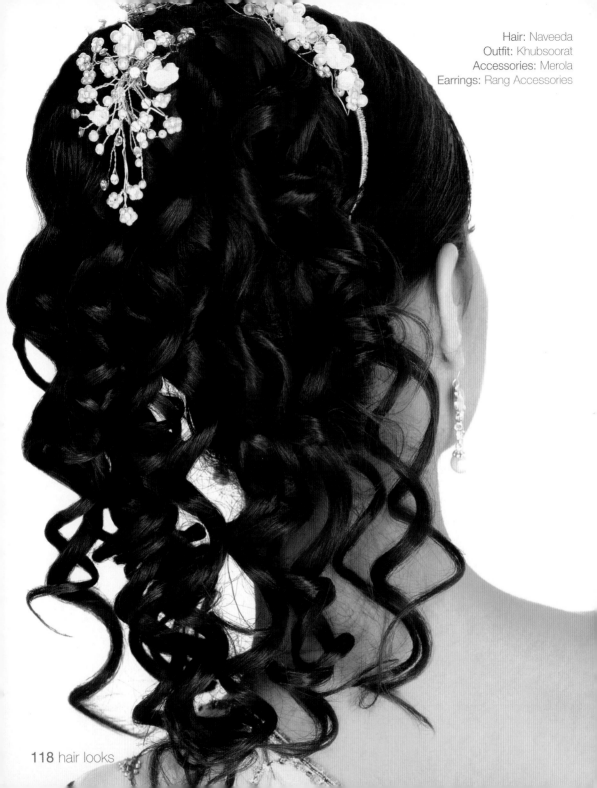

Hair: Naveeda
Outfit: Khubsoorat
Accessories: Merola
Earrings: Rang Accessories

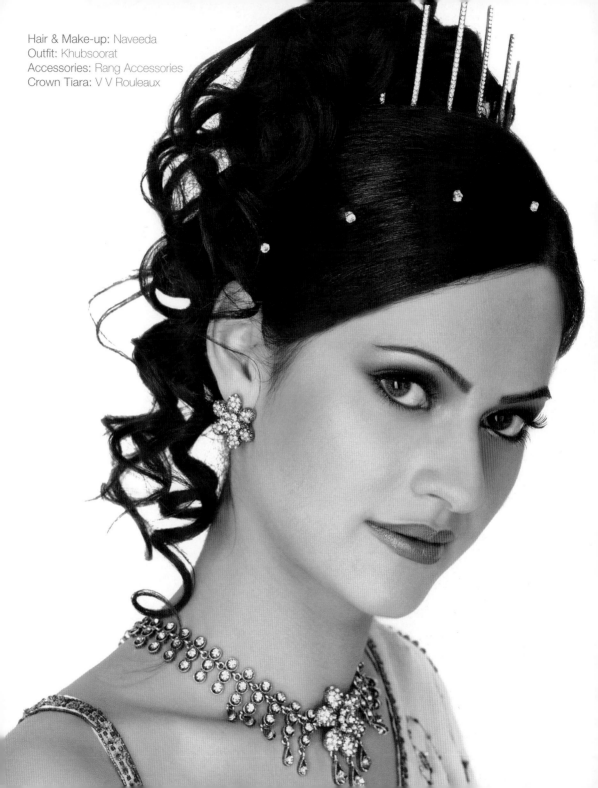

Hair & Make-up: Naveeda
Outfit: Khubsoorat
Accessories: Rang Accessories
Crown Tiara: V V Rouleaux

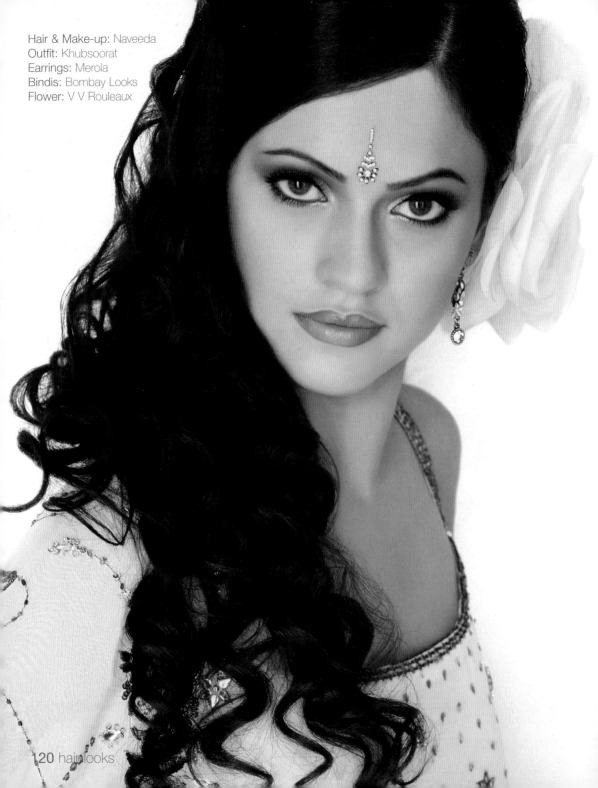

Hair & Make-up: Naveeda
Outfit: Khubsoorat
Earrings: Merola
Bindis: Bombay Looks
Flower: V V Rouleaux

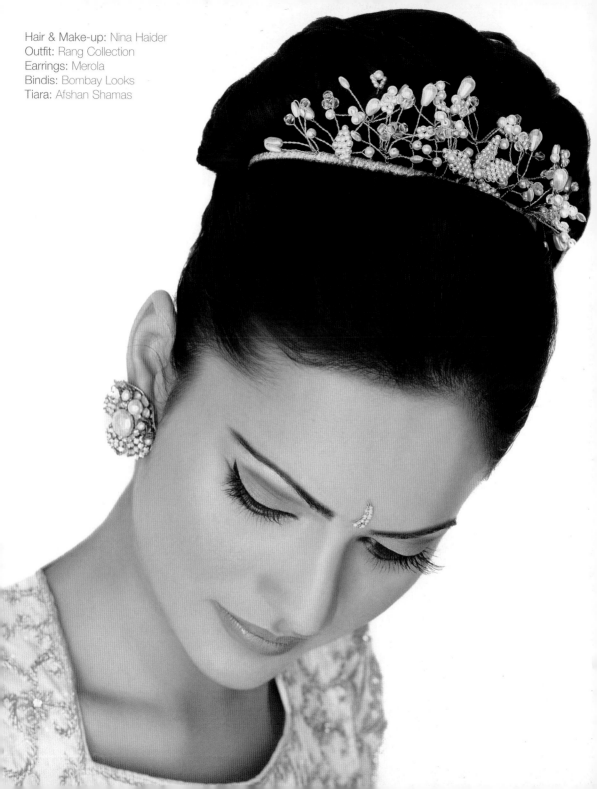

Hair & Make-up: Nina Haider
Outfit: Rang Collection
Earrings: Merola
Bindis: Bombay Looks
Tiara: Afshan Shamas

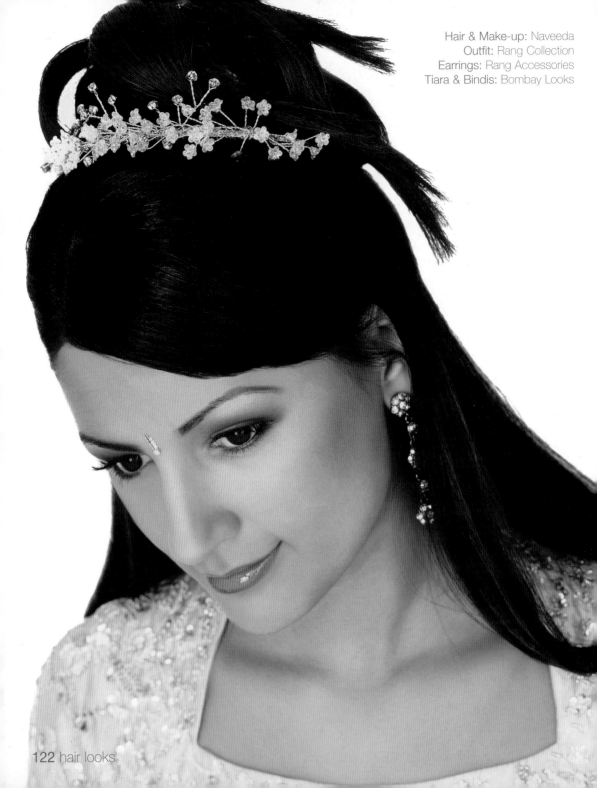

Hair & Make-up: Naveeda
Outfit: Rang Collection
Earrings: Rang Accessories
Tiara & Bindis: Bombay Looks

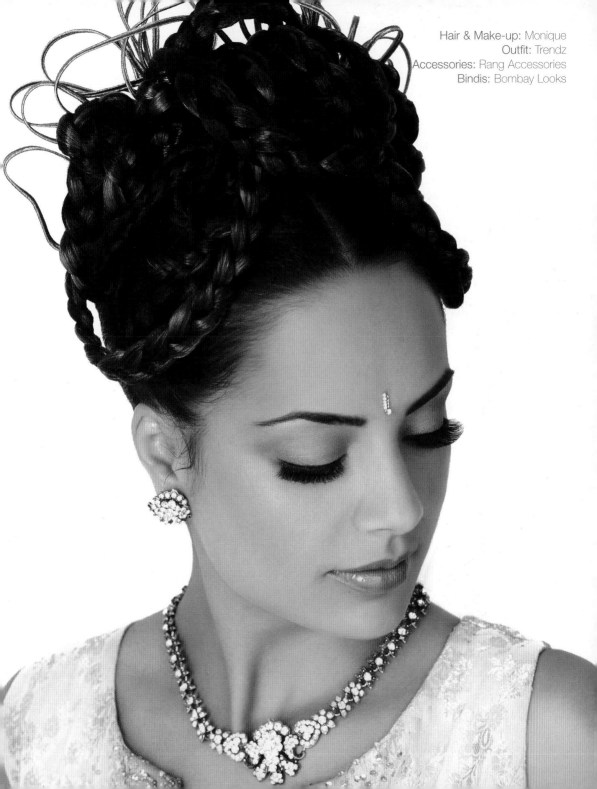

Hair & Make-up: Monique
Outfit: Trendz
Accessories: Rang Accessories
Bindis: Bombay Looks

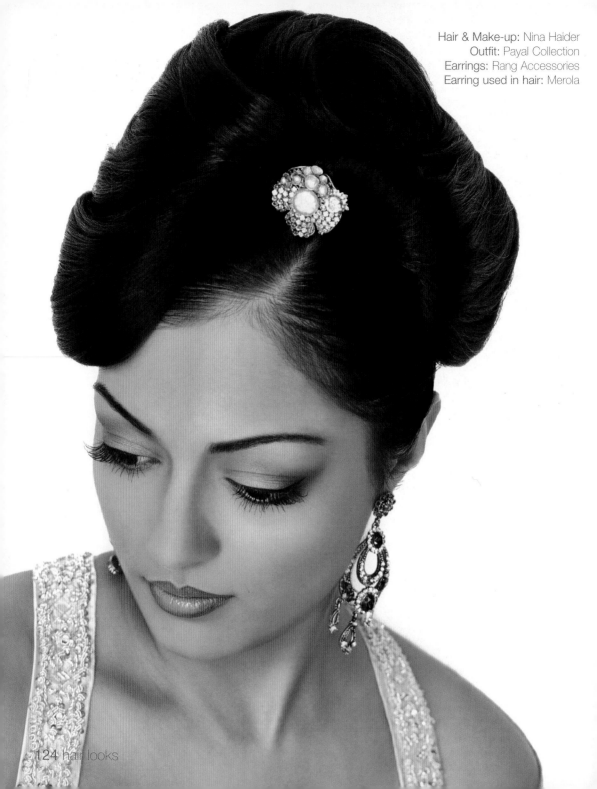

Hair & Make-up: Nina Haider
Outfit: Payal Collection
Earrings: Rang Accessories
Earring used in hair: Merola

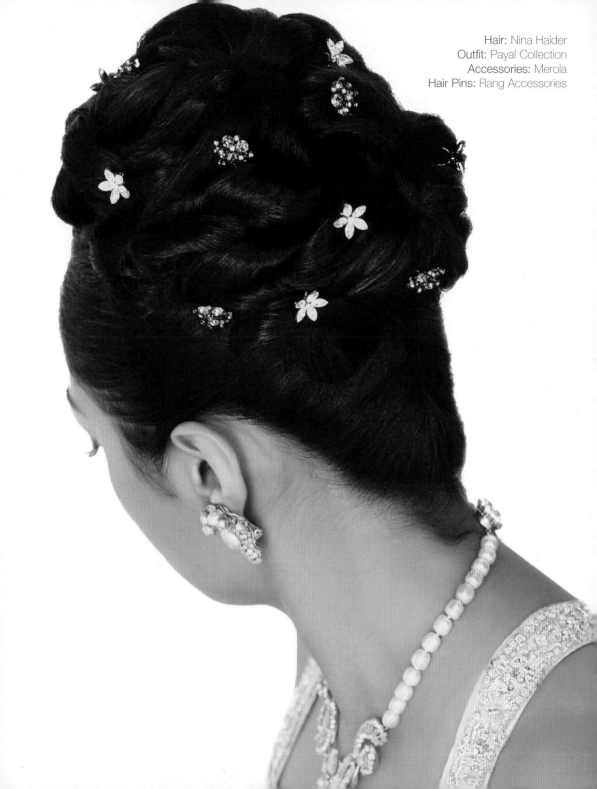

Hair: Nina Haider
Outfit: Payal Collection
Accessories: Merola
Hair Pins: Rang Accessories

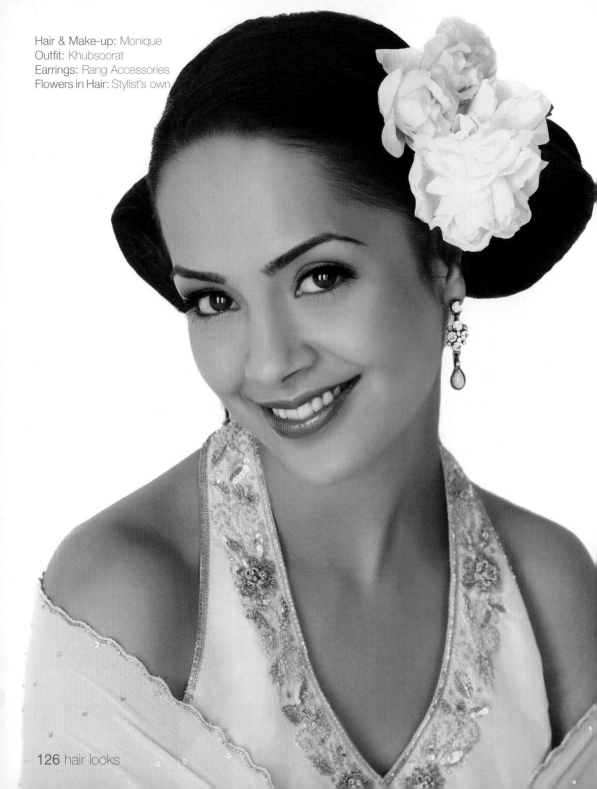

Hair & Make-up: Monique
Outfit: Khubsoorat
Earrings: Rang Accessories
Flowers in Hair: Stylist's own

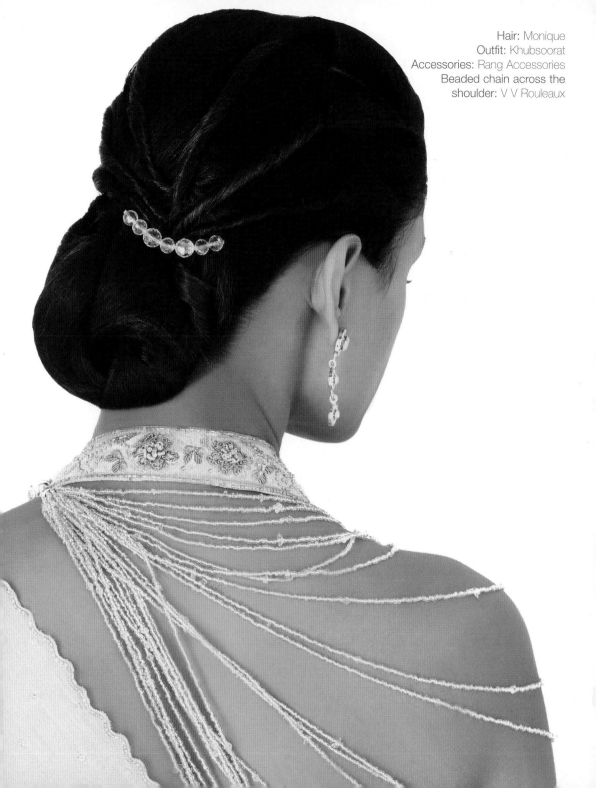

Hair: Monique
Outfit: Khubsoorat
Accessories: Rang Accessories
Beaded chain across the
shoulder: V V Rouleaux

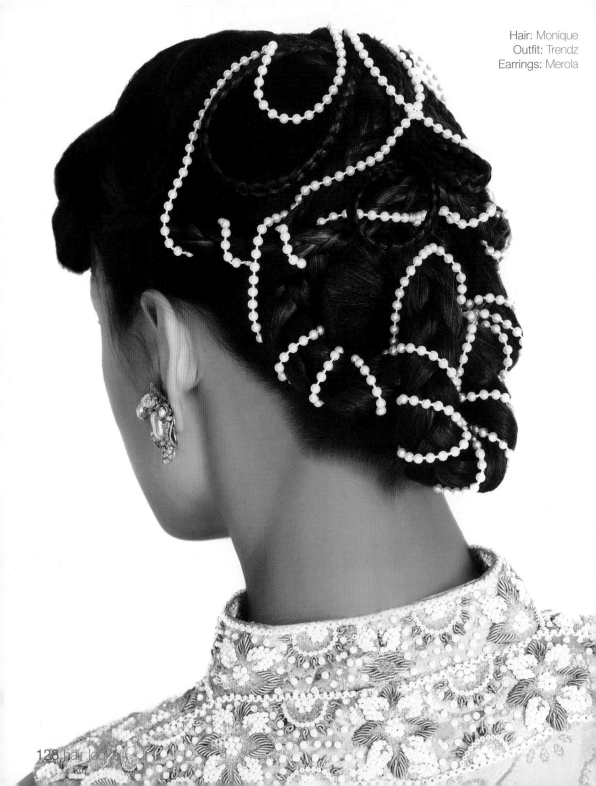

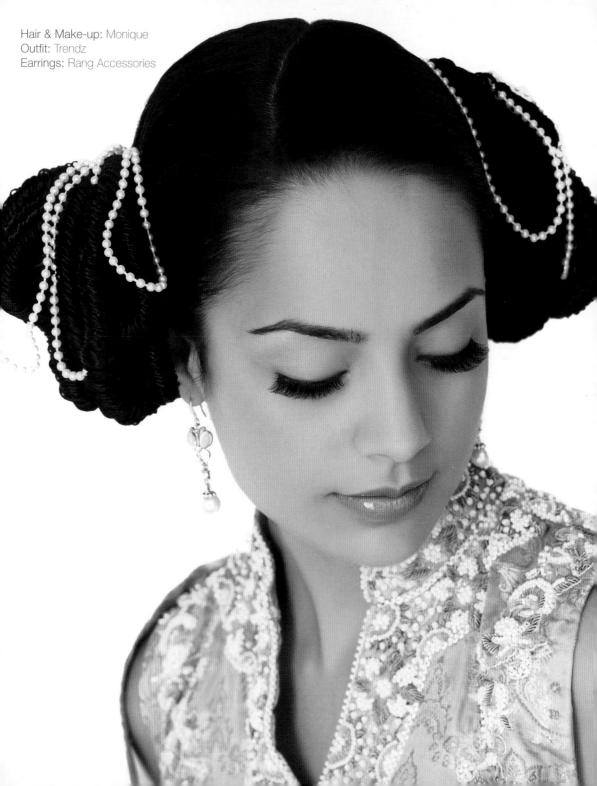

Hair & Make-up: Monique
Outfit: Trendz
Earrings: Rang Accessories

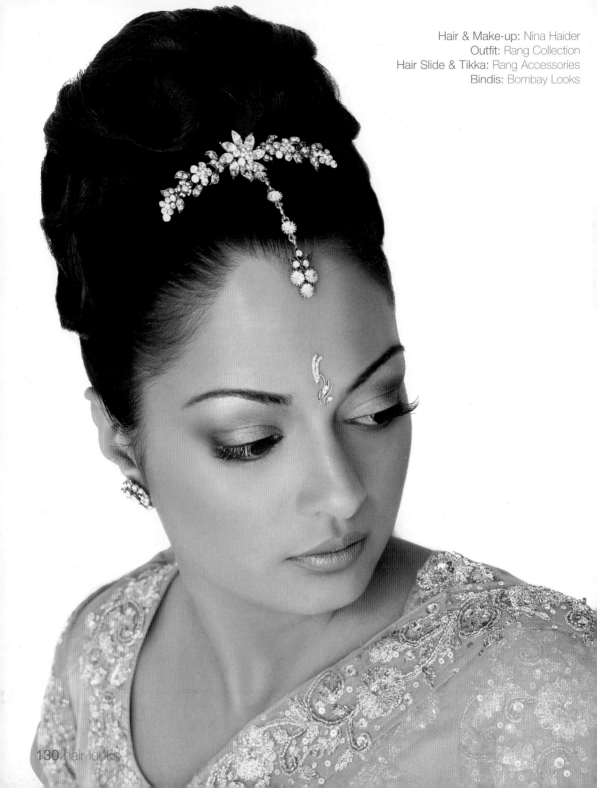

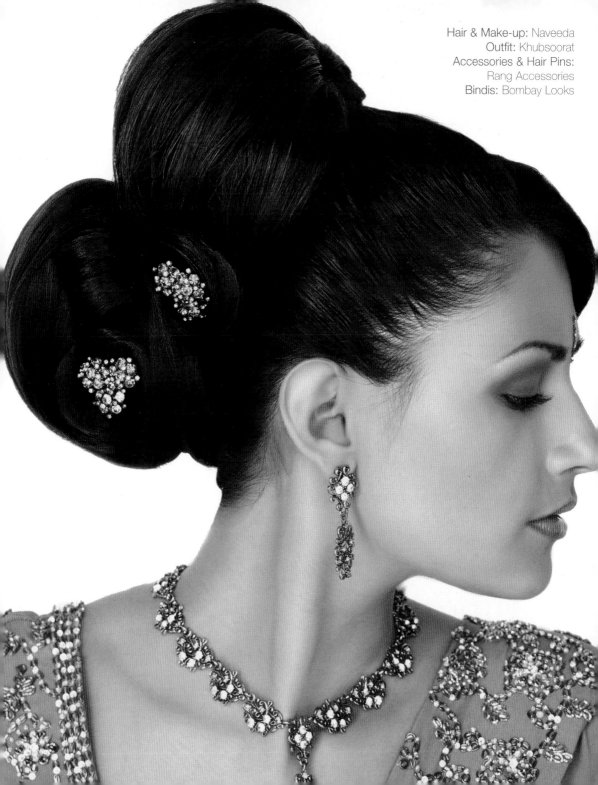

Hair & Make-up: Naveeda
Outfit: Khubsoorat
Accessories & Hair Pins:
Rang Accessories
Bindis: Bombay Looks

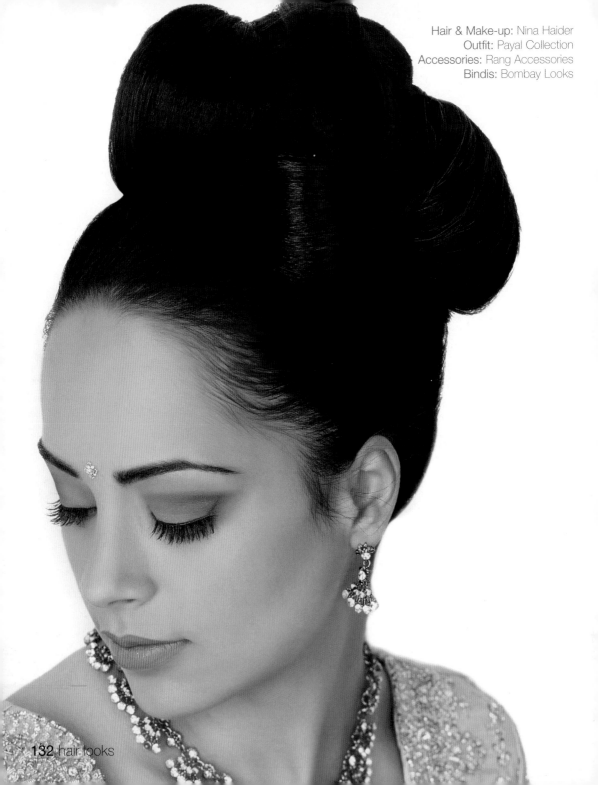

Hair & Make-up: Nina Haider
Outfit: Payal Collection
Accessories: Rang Accessories
Bindis: Bombay Looks

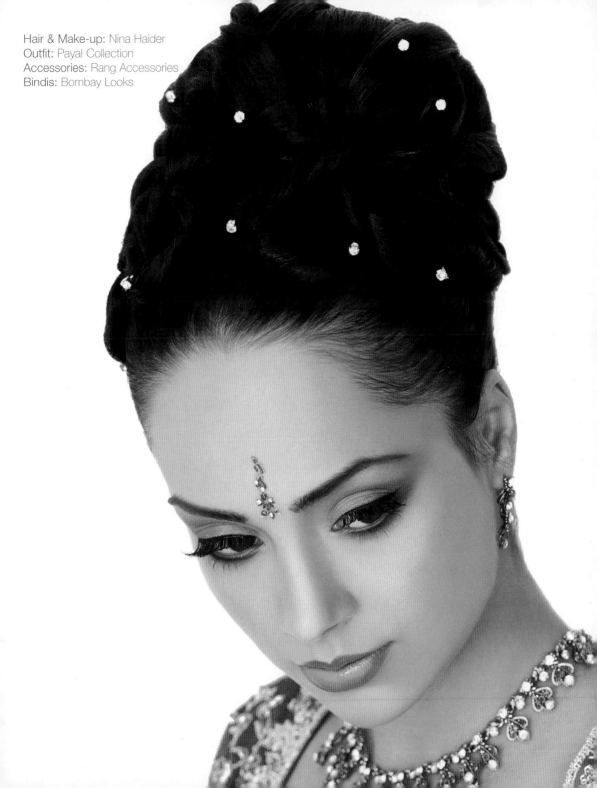

Hair & Make-up: Nina Haider
Outfit: Payal Collection
Accessories: Rang Accessories
Bindis: Bombay Looks

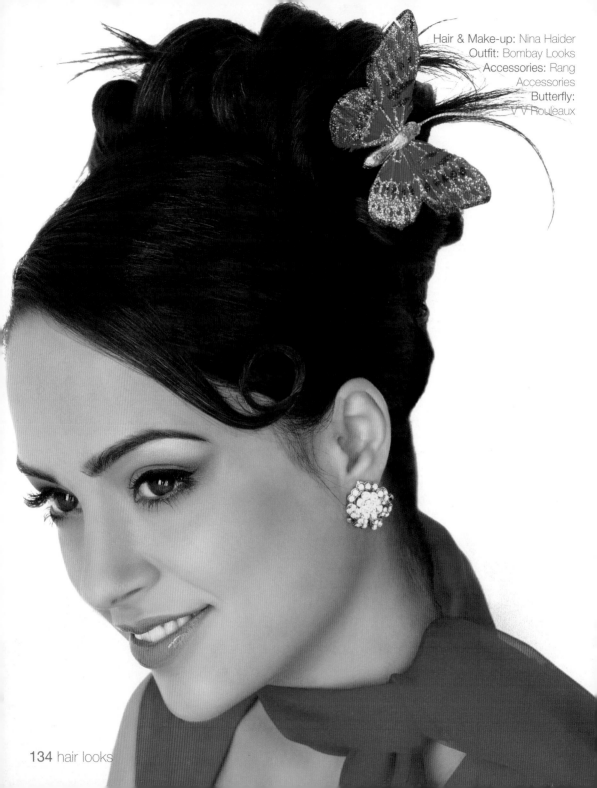

Hair & Make-up: Nina Haider
Outfit: Bombay Looks
Accessories: Rang
Accessories
Butterfly:
V V Rouleaux

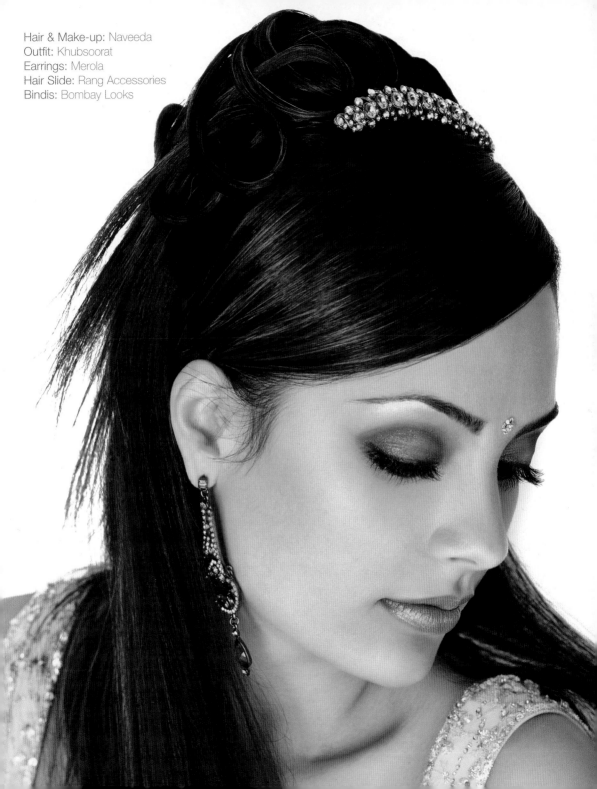

Hair & Make-up: Naveeda
Outfit: Khubsoorat
Earrings: Merola
Hair Slide: Rang Accessories
Bindis: Bombay Looks

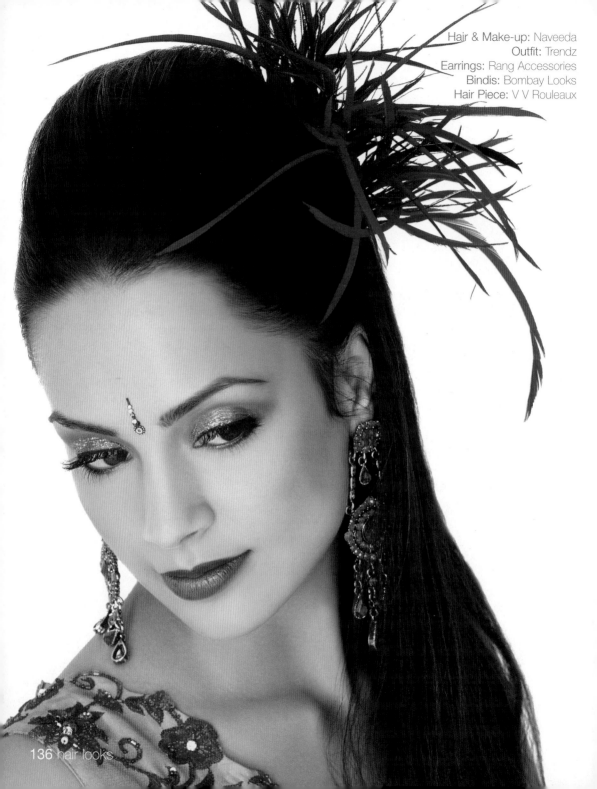

Hair & Make-up: Naveeda
Outfit: Trendz
Earrings: Rang Accessories
Bindis: Bombay Looks
Hair Piece: V V Rouleaux

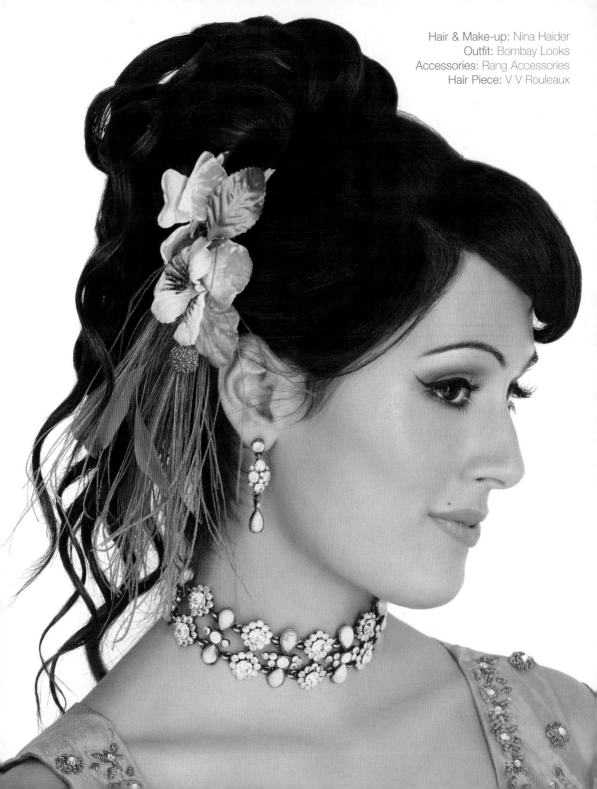

Hair & Make-up: Nina Haider
Outfit: Bombay Looks
Accessories: Rang Accessories
Hair Piece: V V Rouleaux

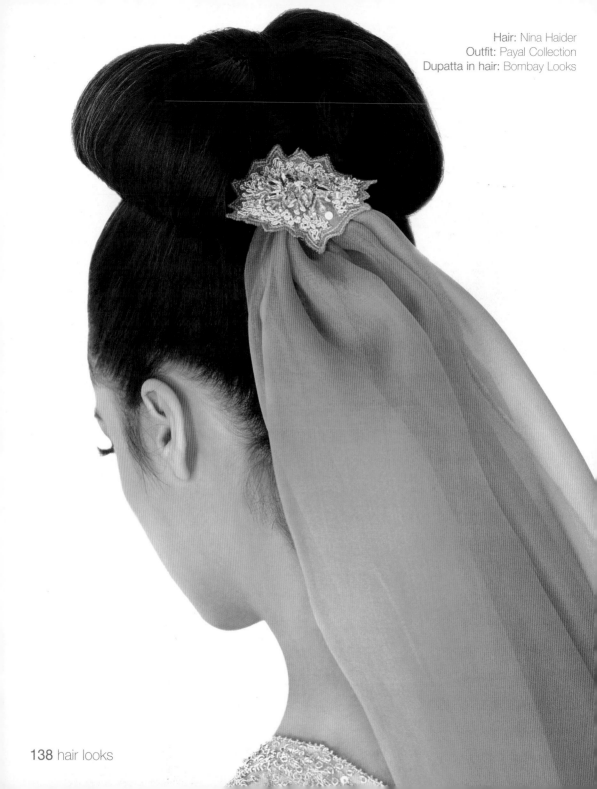

Hair: Nina Haider
Outfit: Payal Collection
Dupatta in hair: Bombay Looks

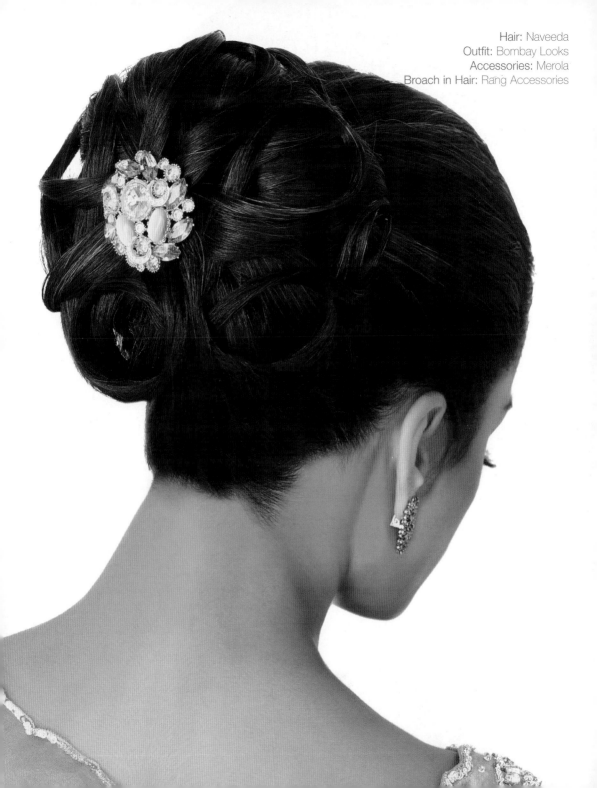

Hair: Naveeda
Outfit: Bombay Looks
Accessories: Merola
Broach in Hair: Rang Accessories

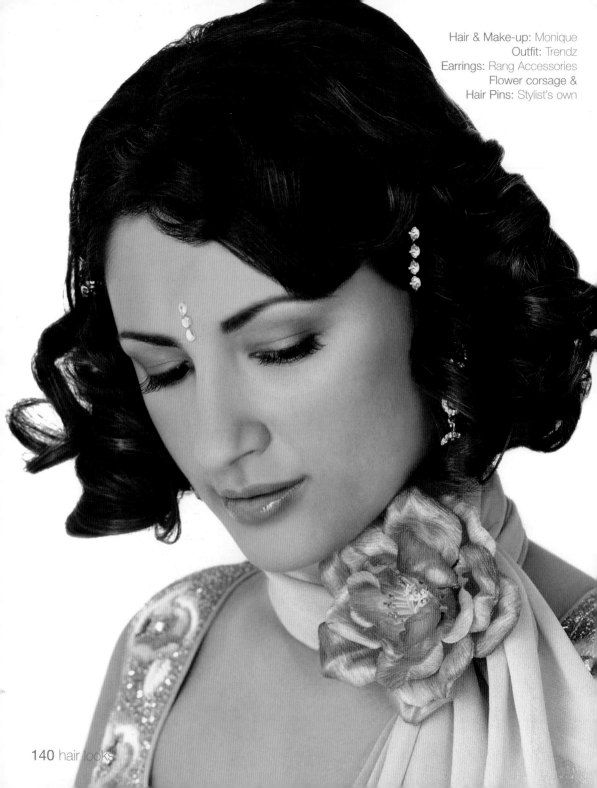

Hair & Make-up: Monique
Outfit: Trendz
Earrings: Rang Accessories
Flower corsage &
Hair Pins: Stylist's own

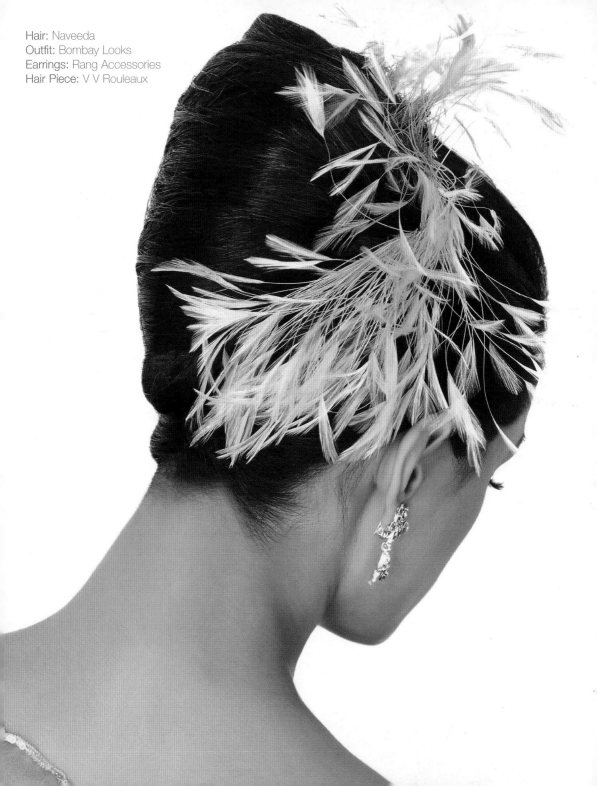

Hair: Naveeda
Outfit: Bombay Looks
Earrings: Rang Accessories
Hair Piece: V V Rouleaux

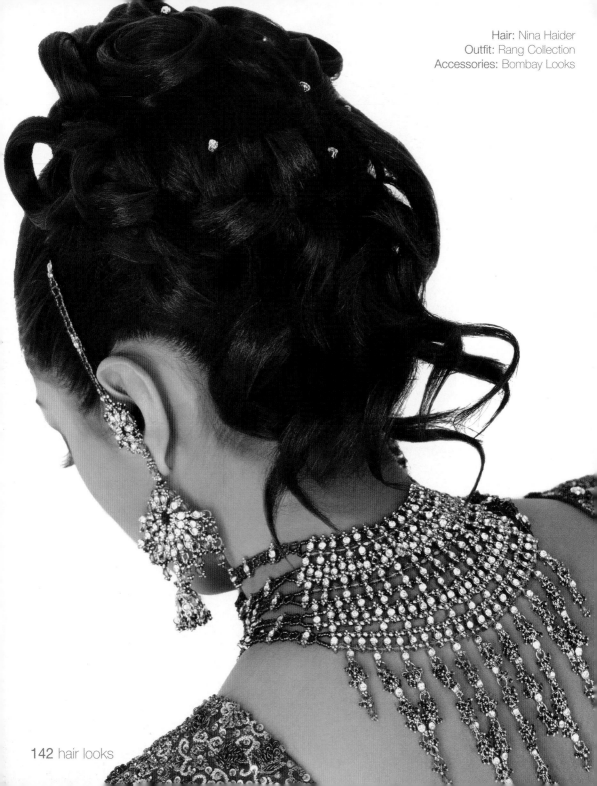

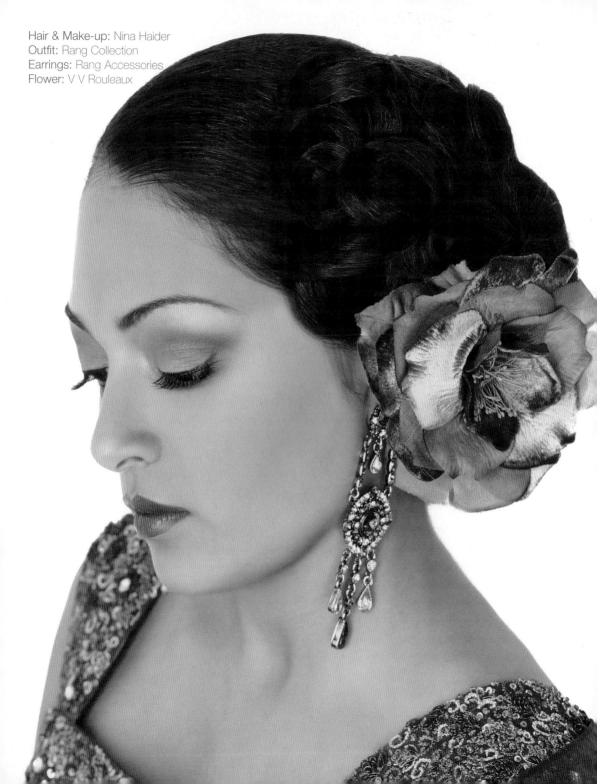

Hair & Make-up: Nina Haider
Outfit: Rang Collection
Earrings: Rang Accessories
Flower: V V Rouleaux

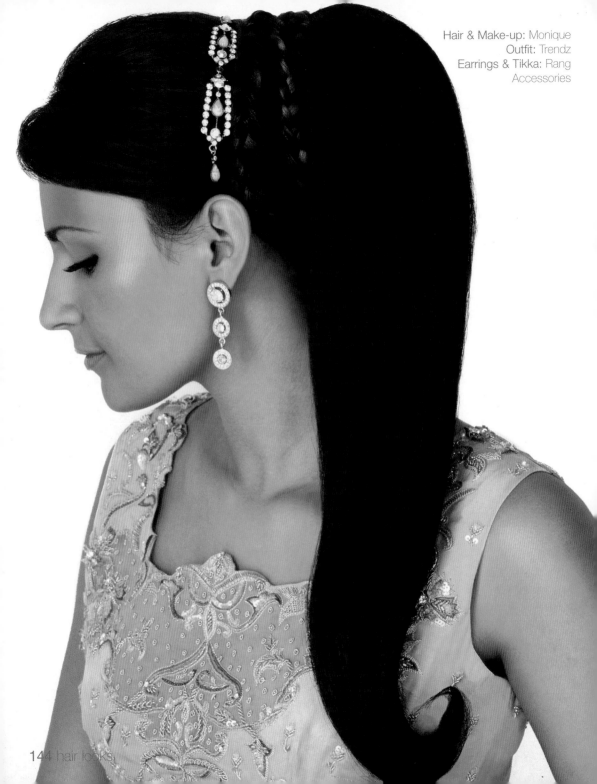

Hair & Make-up: Monique
Outfit: Trendz
Earrings & Tikka: Rang
Accessories

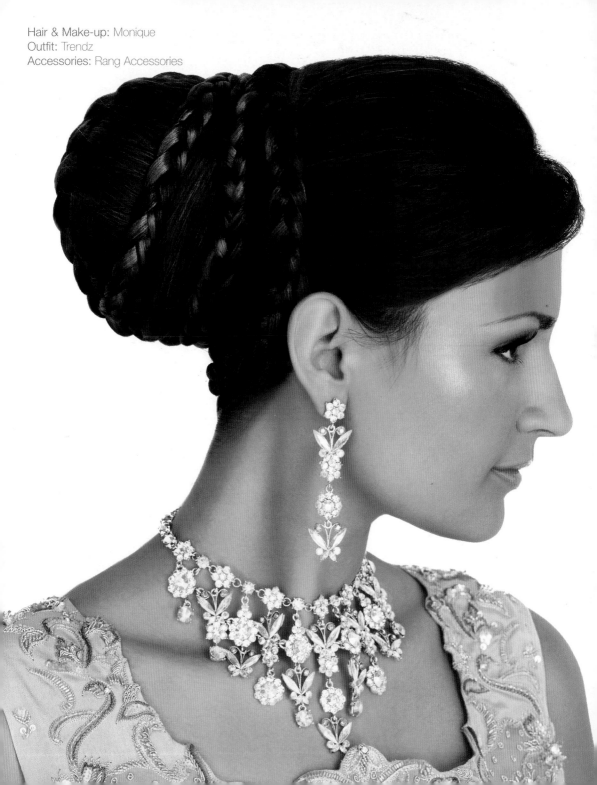

Hair & Make-up: Monique
Outfit: Trendz
Accessories: Rang Accessories

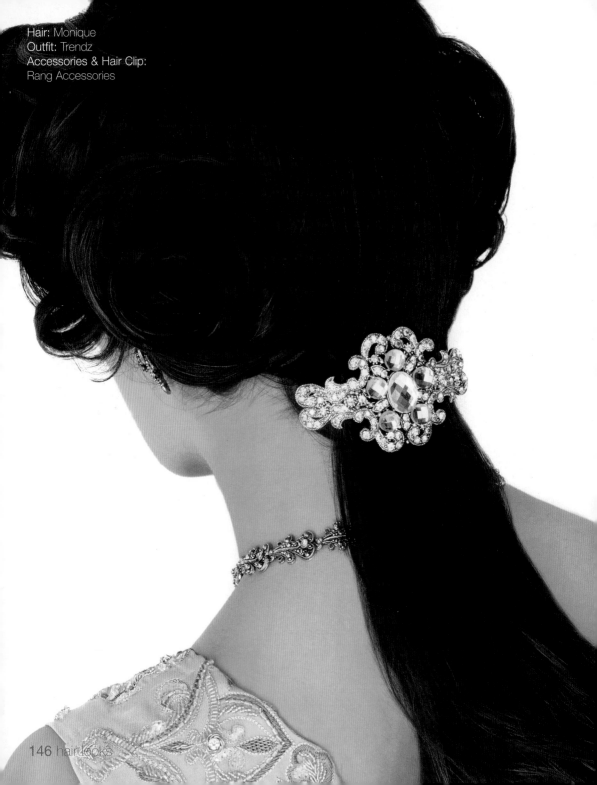

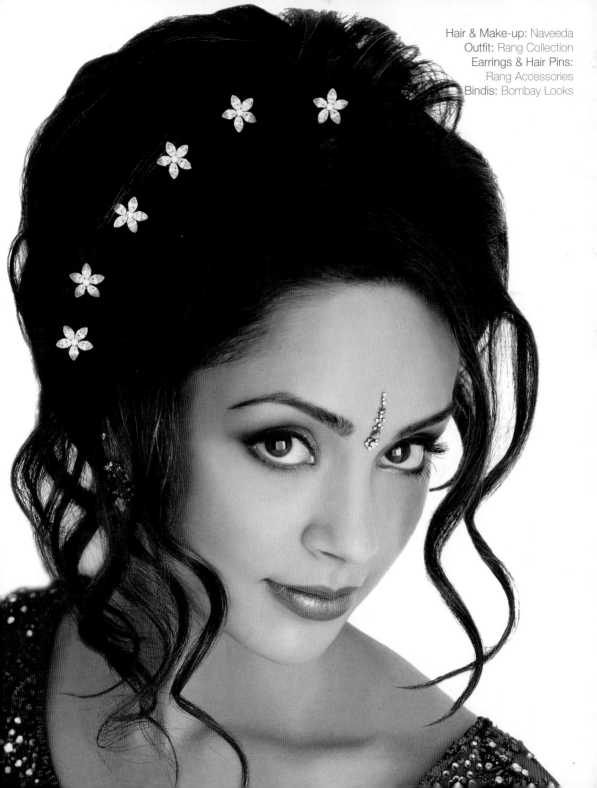

Hair & Make-up: Naveeda
Outfit: Rang Collection
Earrings & Hair Pins:
Rang Accessories
Bindis: Bombay Looks

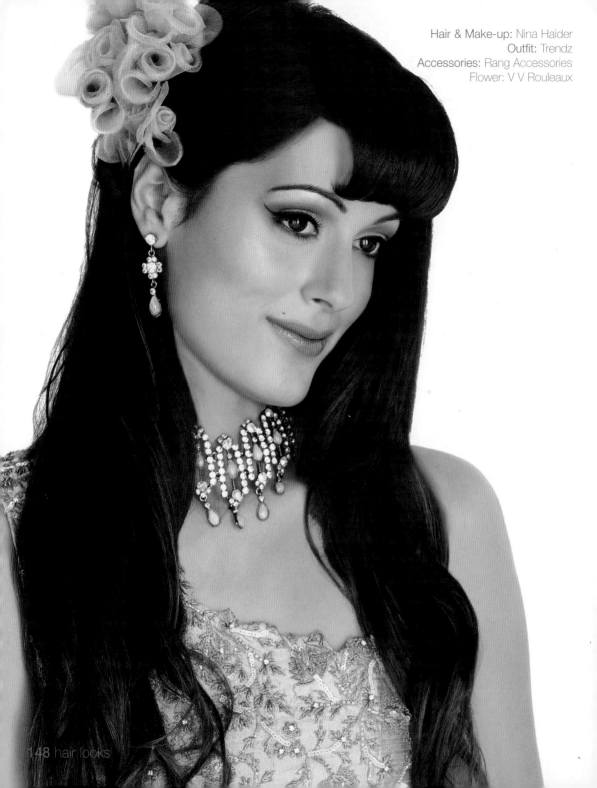

Hair & Make-up: Nina Haider
Outfit: Trendz
Accessories: Rang Accessories
Flower: V V Rouleaux

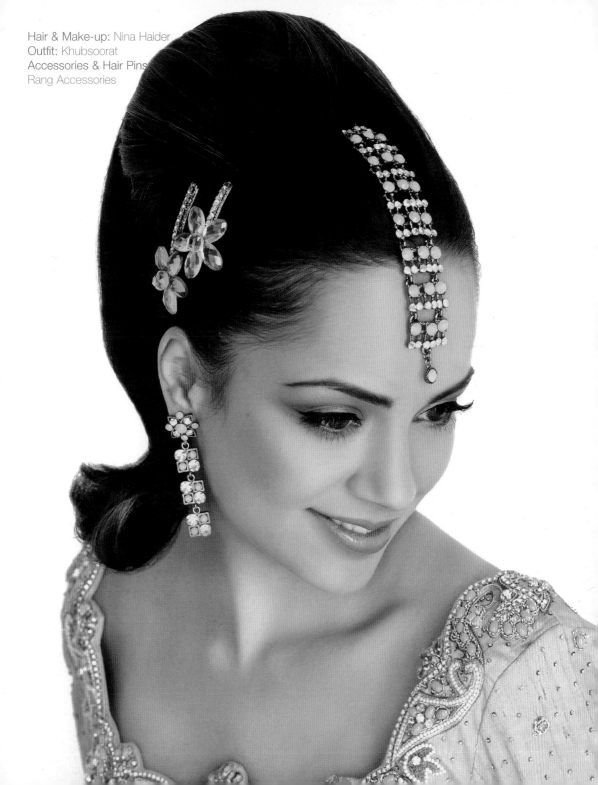

Hair & Make-up: Nina Haider
Outfit: Khubsoorat
Accessories & Hair Pins
Rang Accessories

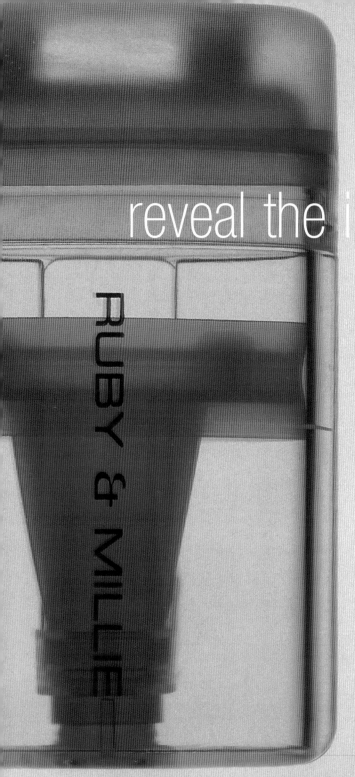

reveal the inner you...

RUBY & MILLIE

available at larger boots stores

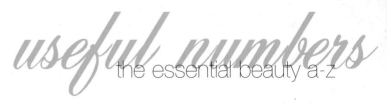
the ultimate make-up artists

Have you ever imagined having a top make-up artist transform you into a vision of bridal beauty? Have you ever imagined having your hair and make-up done by the very celebrity artists that created the gorgeous looks on these pages? Well, here's your chance... just remember to tell them how much you loved their work!

Naveeda 07958 635 857   www.naveeda.com

Nina Haider 07957 252 524

Monique Lagnerius 07970 447 724

the best beauty & hair products

Avon	0845 345 8444
Becca @ Space NK	020 7299 4999
Benefit	0901 113 0001
Chanel	020 7493 3836
Clinique	01730 232566
Elizabeth Arden	www.elizabetharden.com
Garnier Fructis	www.garnierfructis.com
Givenchy	020 7563 8800
Guerlain	01932 233874
Iman	www.imanbeauty.com
Kiehl's	020 7734 1234
Lancôme	www.lancome.co.uk
L'Oreal tecni-art	0800 072 6699
Mac	020 7534 9222
Nars	020 7299 4999
Paul Mitchell	01296 390 590
Revlon	0800 085 2715
Rimmel	www.rimmellondon.com
RMK	020 7259 5669
Ruby & Millie	www.boots.com
Stila	01730 232566
Tigi	0870 330 0955
Umberto Giannini	07000 862 3786
VO5	www.vo5.com
Vincent Longo	www.vincentlongo.com

fabulous fashion

Bombay Looks
164 Green Street, London, E7
020 8471 2444
185 Ilford Lane, Ilford, Essex
020 8478 3882
87e Belgrave Road, Leicester
0116 261 0241

Khubsoorat
117 Green Street, London, E7
0208475 0037
113 Broadway, Hickville, New York, 11801
001 516 935 8404

Payal Collection
275a Green Street, London, E7
020 8586 0161

Rang Collection
PO Box 786, Hornchurch, Essex, RM11
01708 345 786

Trendz
71 Green Street, London, E7
020 85481 786

amazing accessories

Afshan Shamas   020 8530 4464
(by appointment only)

Bombay Looks   see fashion for details

Merola   020 7351 9338

Rang Accessories   01708 345 786

V V Rouleaux   020 7730 3125

perfect pictures

Alexandre Pichon   07990 975 425

remember to mention the asian bridal look book when calling!

beauty diary
create your look

occasion: _____ date: _____

page reference from the asian bridal look book for:					
options	1	2	3	4	5
make up					
hair					

notes: _____

_____

_____

_____

_____

_____

_____

_____

_____

_____

_____

occasion: _____ date: _____

page reference from the asian bridal look book for:					
options	1	2	3	4	5
make up					
hair					

notes:
_____
_____
_____
_____
_____
_____
_____
_____
_____
_____
_____
_____

beauty diary
create your look

occasion: _____ date: _____

page reference from the asian bridal look book for:					
options	1	2	3	4	5
make up					
hair					

notes:
_____
_____
_____
_____
_____
_____
_____
_____
_____
_____

occasion: _____ date: _____

page reference from the asian bridal look book for:					
options	1	2	3	4	5
make up					
hair					

notes:
_____
_____
_____
_____
_____
_____
_____
_____
_____
_____
_____
_____

acknowledgements
we would like to thank...

"I wouldn't be where I am today had it not been for the love and support of my husband, mehtab, and my children, omar & asim. They truly are the inspiration behind what I do."
naveeda

"I would like to thank my son humza haider, my late husband haider nawaz and my mother for their kind support and blessings."
nina haider

"Special thanks to john hughes and dev lyall, to whom without their support and dedication, this book would not have been possible. Also to our parents; surinder & bimla lyall, mahendra & vimla bharadia, for their continuous love and guidance."
kiran and nilpa

We would also like to thank the following

aishwariya rai, aisha shahid, alexandre & karen pichon, alexandra elischer, ali panchoo, amrit, aruna, baljit dhuper, beena nadeem, caroline at pure pr, charlotte moore, confetti, dave essex, fnik pr, fuad omar, gurmukh manchanda, hammasa, harriet at purple pr, ifraz ahmed, jon matthews, kim, kiran & rupert verdi, mandeep, mani & mickey at khubsoorat, martin, monique, mr & mrs v padhiar, nadia at rang accessories, namita asthana, naveeda & mehtab, navreet jhutti, nazia at rang collection, neelam & asad at trendz, nina haider, pamla kalha, paresh & subhash at bombay looks, pirvinder bansel, priya lyall, rashpal parmar, richard miller, ruby hammer & millie kendall, ruple vaid, saheda adia, sajnit bhandal, sanjay dhir, sarwar ahmed, sawan bharadia, shihab salim, steve austin, suresh at payal collection, tamsin at coty inc, trinaina bharij, vanessa srao, venisha padhiar, vin nandra, vinny & ranjana mitra, will sweet, zulika bibi

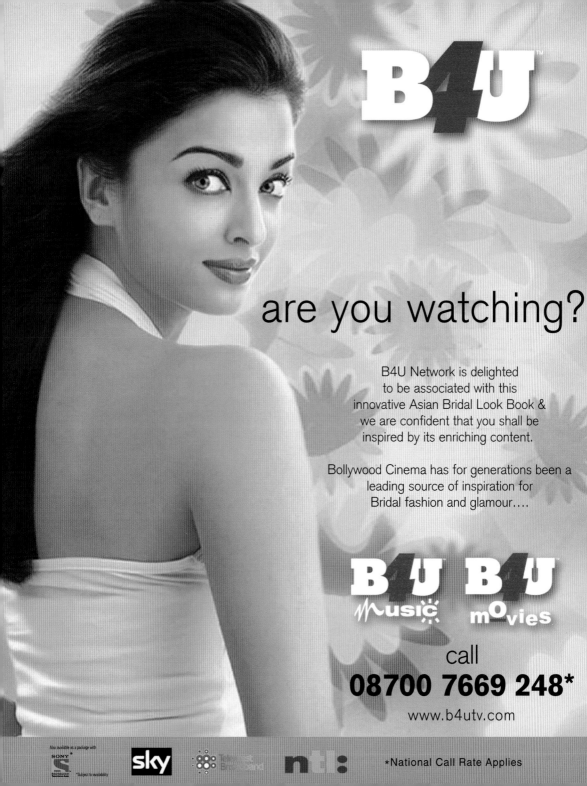

index
colour guide